INTERNAL MEDICINE

Mastering The Boards and Clinical Examinations

INFECTIOUS DISEASES

A.B.R. Thomson

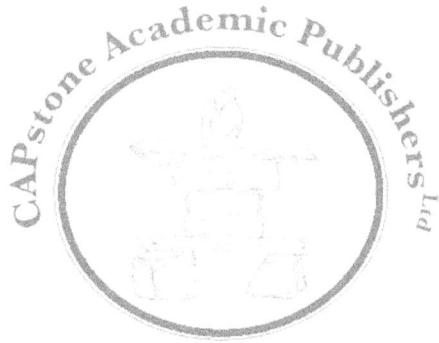

CAPstone (Canadian Academic Publishers Ltd) is a not-for-profit company dedicated to the use of the power of education for the betterment of all persons everywhere.

"The Democratization of Knowledge"

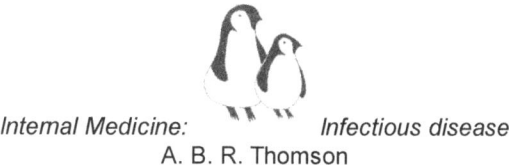

Internal Medicine: Infectious disease
A. B. R. Thomson

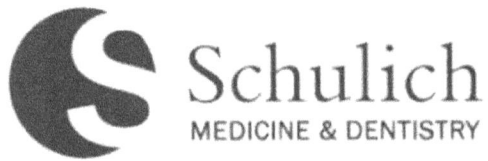

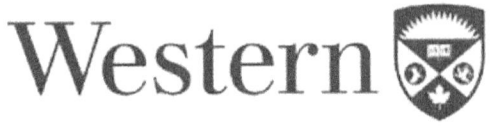

THE WESTERN WAY

Internal Medicine: *Infectious disease*
A. B. R. Thomson

Table of Contents

Disclaimer

The primary purpose of this publication is education. The author, editor and publisher acknowledge that the development of new material opens to way for possible errors – what is correct today might not be the standard of care tomorrow. Readers are advised to ensure that the doses of drugs which they use are in compliance with their country's product information, and that the use of any therapeutic agent, be it a pharmaceutical or a technology, should be guided by local guidelines. There is often a wide diversity of professional opinion, and guidelines from one country are not always congruent with another.

The author, editor and publisher do not guarantee the safety, reliability, accuracy, completeness or usefulness of this material.

They disclaim any and all liability for damage and claims that may result from the use of information, publications, technologies, products, and for series provided in this publication.

We have made every attempt to trace the holders of copyright for material reproduced in this book. If by some oversight we have omitted a copyright holder, please contact us.

Thank you

Alan Thomson

Internal Medicine: *Infectious diseases*
A. B. R. Thomson

Mastering The Boards And The Canmed Objectives

Medical expert

The discussion of complex cases provides the participants with an opportunity to comment on additional focused history and physical examination. They would provide a complete and organized assessment. Participants are encouraged to identify key features, and they develop an approach to problem-solving.

The case discussions, as well as the discussion of cases around a diagnostic imaging, pathological or endoscopic base provides the means for the candidate to establish an appropriate management plan based on the best available evidence to clinical practice. Throughout, an attempt is made to develop strategies for diagnosis and development of clinical reasoning skills.

Communicator

The participants demonstrate their ability to communicate their knowledge, clinical findings, and management plan in a respectful, concise and interactive manner. When the participants play the role of examiners, they demonstrate their ability to listen actively and effectively, to ask questions in an open-ended manner, and to provide constructive, helpful feedback in a professional and non-intimidating manner.

Collaborator

The participants use the "you have a green consult card" technique of answering questions as fast as they are able, and then to interact with another health professional participant to move forward the discussion and problem solving. This helps the participants to build upon what they have already learned about the importance of collegial interaction.

Manager

The participants are provided with assignments in advance of the three day GI Practice Review. There is much work for them to complete before as well as afterwards, so they learn to manage their time effectively, and to complete the assigned tasks proficiently and on time. They learn to work in teams to achieve answers from small group participation, and then to share this with other small group participants through effective delegation of work. Some of the material they must access demands that they use information technology effectively to access information that will help to facilitate the delineation of adequately broad differential diagnoses, as well as rational and cost effective management plans.

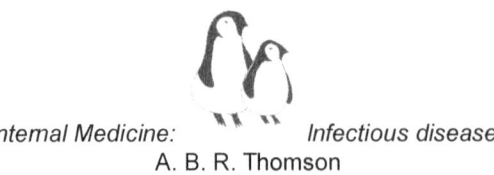

Internal Medicine: *Infectious diseases*
A. B. R. Thomson

Health advocate

In the answering of the questions and case discussions, the participants are required to consider the risks, benefits, and costs and impacts of investigations and therapeutic alliances upon the patient and their loved ones.

Scholar

By committing to the pre- and post-study requirements, plus the intense three day active learning Practice Review with colleagues is a demonstration of commitment to personal education. Through the interactive nature of the discussions and the use of the "green consult card", they reinforce their previous learning of the importance of collaborating and helping one another to learn.

Professional

The participants are coached how to interact verbally in a professional setting, being straightforward, clear and helpful. They learn to be honest when they cannot answer questions, make a diagnosis, or advance a management plan. They learn how to deal with aggressive or demotivated colleagues, how to deal with knowledge deficits, how to speculate on a missing knowledge byte by using first principals and deductive reasoning. In a safe and supportive setting they learn to seek and accept advice, to acknowledge awareness of personal limitations, and to give and take 360° feedback.

Knowledge

The basic science aspects of gastroenterology are considered in adequate detail to understand the mechanisms of disease, and the basis of investigations and treatment. In this way, the participants respect the importance of an adequate foundation in basic sciences, the basics of the design of clinical research studies to provide an evidence-based approach, the designing of clinical research studies to provide an evidence-based approach, the relevance of their management plans being patient-focused, and the need to add "compassionate" to the Three C's of Medical Practice: competent, caring and compassionate.

"They may forget what you said, but they will never forget how you made them feel."

Carl W. Buechner, on teaching

"With competence, care for the patient. With compassion, care about the person."

Alan B. R. Thomson, on being a physician.

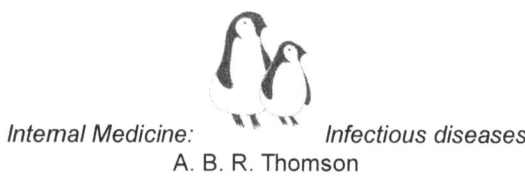

Internal Medicine: *Infectious diseases*
A. B. R. Thomson

Prologue

HREs, better known as, High Risk Examinations. After what is often two decades of study, sacrifice, long hours, dedication, ambition and drive, we who have chosen Internal Medicine, and possibly through this a subspecialty, have a HRE, the [Boards] Royal College Examinations. We have been evaluated almost daily by the sadly subjective preceptor based assessments, and now we face the fierce, competitive, winner-take-all objective testing through multiple choice questions (MCQs), and for some the equally challenging OSCE, the objective standardized clinical examination. Well we know that in the real life of providing competent, caring and compassionate care as physicians, as internists, that a patient is neither a MCQ or an OSCE. These examinations are to be passed, a process with which we may not necessarily agree. Yet this is the game in which we have thus far invested over half of our youthful lives. So let us know the rules, follow the rules, work with the rules, and succeed. So that we may move on to do what we have been trained to do, do what we may long to do, care for our patients.

The process by which we study for clinical examinations is so is different than for the MCQs: not trivia, but an approach to the big picture, with thoughtful and reasoned deduction towards a diagnosis. Not looking for the answer before us, but understanding the subtle aspects of the directed history and focused physical examination, yielding an informed series of hypotheses, a differential diagnosis to direct investigations of the highly sophisticated laboratory and imaging procedures now available to those who can wait, or pay.

This book provides clinically relevant questions of the process of taking a history and performing a physical examination, with sections on Useful background, and where available, evidence-based performance characteristics of the rendering of our clinical skills. Just for fun are included "So you want to be a such-and-such specialist!" to remind us that one if the greatest strengths we can possess to survive in these times, is to smile and even to laugh at ourselves.

Sincerely,

Alan Thomson
Emeritus Distinguished University Professor, University of Alberta

Adjunct Professor, Western University

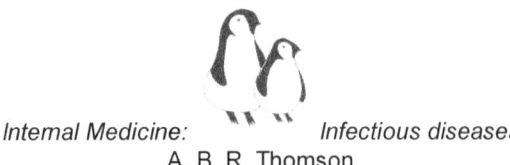

Internal Medicine: *Infectious diseases*
A. B. R. Thomson

Dedication

To My Family

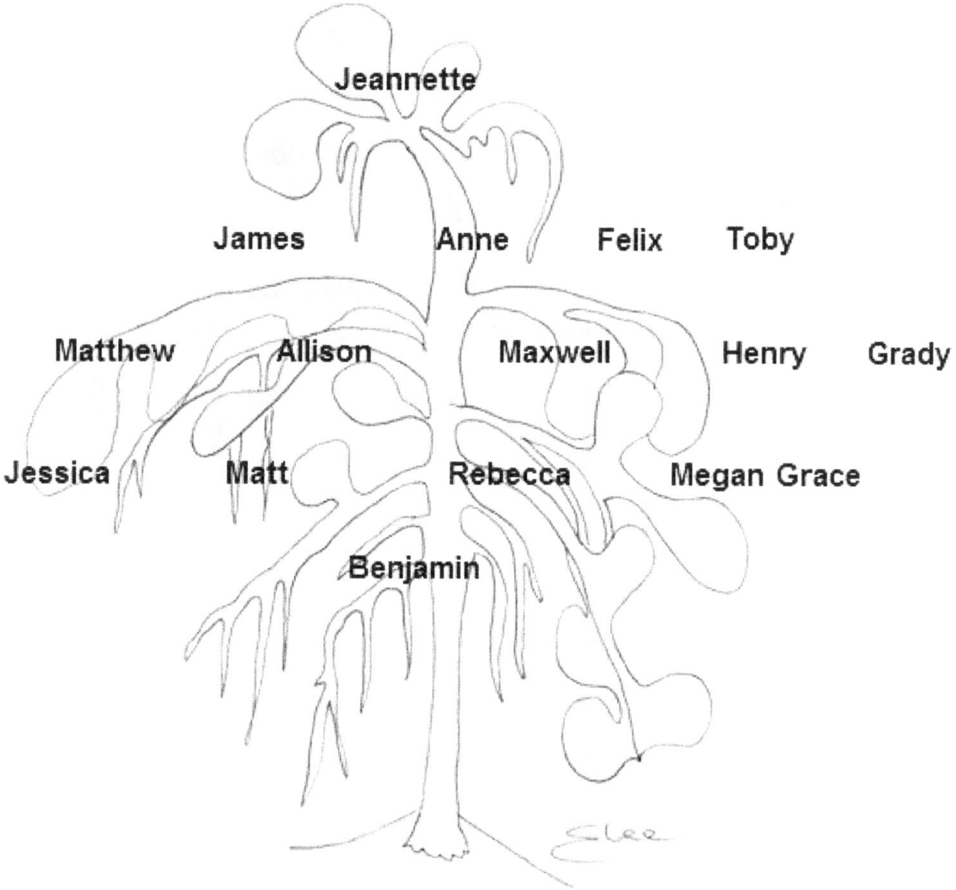

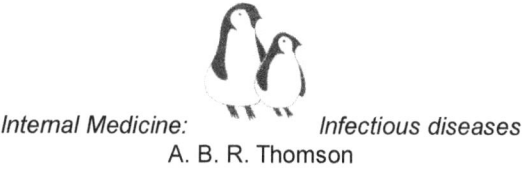

Jeannette

James   Anne   Felix   Toby

Matthew   Allison   Maxwell   Henry   Grady

Jessica   Matt   Rebecca   Megan Grace

Benjamin

For your support, caring and love

During these challenging years

And always.

Mark 15:34

Luke 23:34

Domenichino 16:41

Corinthians 1:13

Internal Medicine: *Infectious diseases*
A. B. R. Thomson

Acknowledgements

Patience and patients go hand in hand. So also does the interlocking of young and old, love and justice, equality and fairness. No author can have thoughts transformed into words, no teacher can make ideas become behaviour and wisdom and art, without those special people who turn our minds to the practical - of getting the job done!

Thank you, Naiyana and Duen for translating those terrible scribbles, called my handwriting, into the still magical legibility of the electronic age. Thank you, Sarah, for your creativity and hard work.

My most sincere and heartfelt thanks go to the excellent persons at JP Consulting, and CapStone Academic Publishers. Jessica, you are brilliant, dedicated and caring. Thank you.

When Rebecca, Maxwell, Megan Grace, Henry and Felix ask about their Grandad, I will depend on James and Anne, Matthew and Allison, Jessica and Matt, and Benjamin to be understanding and kind. For what I was trying to say and to do was to make my professional life focused on the three C's - competence, caring, and compassion - and to make my very private personal life dedicated to family - to you all.

Internal Medicine: *Infectious diseases*
A. B. R. Thomson

ARE YOU PREPARING FOR EXAMS IN GASTROENTEROLOGY AND HEPATOLOGY?

See the full range of examination preparation and review publications from CAPstone on Amazon.com

Gastroenterology and Hepatology

First Principles of Gastroenterology and Hepatology in Adults and Children - Volume I – Gastroenterology (ISBN: 978-1494345624)

First Principles of Gastroenterology and Hepatology in Adults and Children - Volume II - Hepatology and Paediatrics (ISBN: 978-1494345501)

Medical Mini Review Series in Gastroenterology and Hepatology: Efficient Refresher for the Busy Clinical Gastroenterologist (ISBN: 978-1502472199)

Medical Mini Review Series in Gastroenterology and Hepatology: Efficient Refresher for the Busy Clinical Gastroenterologist (ISBN: 978-1502472199)

Practice Review in Gastroenterology (ISBN: 978-1500855321)

Practice Review in Hepatopancreatobiliary Diseases and Nutrition (ISBN: 978-1500855734)

Endoscopy and Diagnostic Imaging - Part I: Skin, Nail and Mouth Changes in GI Disease; Esophagus; Stomach; Small intestine; Pancreas (ISBN: 978-1477400579)

Endoscopy and Diagnostic Imaging - Part II: Colon and Hepatobiliary (ISBN: 978-1477400654)

Scientific Basis for Clinical Practice in Gastroenterology and Hepatology (ISBN: 978-1475226645)

The Physiology and Pathophysiology of Gastrointestinal and Hepatopancreaticobiliary Disorders: Preparing for Professional Competence. (ISBN: 978-1500298265)

General Internal Medicine

Achieving Excellence in the OSCE - Part One: Cardiology to Nephrology (ISBN: 978-1475283037)

Achieving Excellence in the OSCE - Part Two: Neurology to Rheumatolgy (ISBN: 978-1475276978)

Mastering the Boards and Clinical Examinations in Internal Medicine, Part I: Cardiology, Endocrinology, Gastroenterology, Hepatology and Nephrology (ISBN: 978-1461024842)

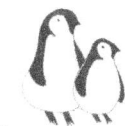

Internal Medicine: *Infectious diseases*
A. B. R. Thomson

Mastering The Boards and Clinical Examinations In Internal Medicine, part II: Neurology, Respirology and Rheumatology (ISBN: 978-1478392736)

Bits and Bytes: Surviving Morning Rounds (ISBN: 978-1478295365)

INFECTIOUS DISEASES

INFECTIOUS DISEASES

BITES AND SCRATCHES

Animal Bites

- ➢ Causes / associations
  - o Staphylococci
  - o Streptococci
  - o Bacteroids
  - o Porphyromonas
  - o Prevotella
  - o Pasteurella multocids
  - o Capnocytophaga
  - o Bartonella henselae (cat-scratch disease)

- ➢ Special clinical points
  - o depth of injury and risk of involving joints / bone
  - o Immune status (of patient)
  - o Previous immunization
    - – Tetanus
    - – Rabies

- ➢ Treatment (including prophylaxis)
  - o No penicillin allergy
    - – Mild
      - ▪ 5 days of amoxicillin-clavulanate
    - – Severe
      - ▪ IV cefoxitin, or carbapenem
  - o Penicillin allergy
    - – Mild
      - ▪ Fluorosquinolone, or
      - ▪ Doxycyclin, or
      - ▪ Trimethoprim-sulfamethoxazole plus clindamycin
    - – Severe
      - ▪ Fluoroquinolone plus clindamycin
      - ▪ Vancomycin
  - o Suspected MRSA
    - – Vancomycin
  - o Duration
    - – Skin 2 wk
    - – Joint 4 wk
    - – Bone 6 wk

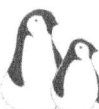

Cat Scratch Disease

- ➤ Cause
  - o Batonella henselae

- ➤ Clinical
  - o 2 d to 2 wk after cat scratch / bite
    - − Erythema
    - − Pustule
    - − Papule
  - o 2 to 3 wk
    - − Lymphadenopathy
    - − Tender
    - − Suppurative

- ➤ Treatment
  - o Self-limited
  - o If infected; azithromycin, short-term
  - o If not infected ,consider prophylaxis with azithromycin

Human Bites

- Give the organism which might infect the person exposed to a human bite.
  - o Anyone who sustains a human bite wound, including a clenched-fist injury, are at risk of developing an infection from the bacterial flora of the mouth, and should be treated. These organisms include
    - − α-hemolytic streptococcus
    - − Staphycoccus
    - − Haemophilus
    - − Eikenella corrodes
    - − B-lactamase producing anaerobes

- ➤ Causes / associations
  - o Oral flora
    - − GABHS
    - − Staphylococci
    - − Haemophilis
    - − Eikenella corrodens

  - o Other infections in blood of attacker
    - − HBV
    - − HCV
    - − HIV
    - − HSV
    - − Syphilis

- ➤ Closed-fist punch
  - o Access for possible involvement of joint, tender, bone

Abbreviation: GABHS, group A beta hemolytic Streptococcus

Internal Medicine: *Infectious disease*
A. B. R. Thomson

In the person who is tolerant to penicillin, amoxicillin-clavulanate is recommended.

- Give the treatment of choice for such a wound in a person who is allergic to penicillin.

    o Clindamycin plus moxifloxacin is recommended

- ➢ Treatment
    - o No evidence of infection
        - – Prophylaxis: amoxicillin-clavulanate, 5 days
    - o Evidence of infection
        - – Cefoxitin or carbopenem
    - o MRSA
        - – Vancomycin

SKIN AND SOFT TISSUE INFECTION (SSTI)

➢ Types

- o Usually
    - – Group A B-hemolytic Streptococci (GABHS)
    - – Staphylococcus
- o Abscess
- o Draining wound
- o Forms of skin and soft tissue infection (SSTI)
    - – Erysipelas
        - ▪ Infection of upper dermis
        - ▪ Legs, arms, face

    - – Cellulitis
        - ▪ Infection of lower dermis, and subcutaneous fat

    - – Abscess
        - ▪ I / D (incision and drainage)
        - ▪ Empiric antibiotics
        - ▪ Lymphangitis
        - ▪ "Peau d'orange"

- o Blood cultures from erysipelas, cellulitis are positive in only ~5%

Please see standard textbooks or reviews such as UptoDate or MKSAP 16, Infectious disease 2012, Table 10, page 13; for cellulitis pathogens with specific behaviours / risk factors

Internal Medicine: *Infectious disease*
A. B. R. Thomson

Purulent Cellulitis

- o Community-Associated Methicillin-Resistant Staphylococcus Aureus (CA-MRSA)

- Give the recommended treatment for non-purulent cellulitis in a patient with fever and leukocytosis, and give the likely organisms against which treatment is directed.

  - o Likely organisms
    - β-hemolytic streptococci
    - CA-MRSA (community-associated methicillin-resistant Staphylococcus aureus)

  - o Recommended antibiotic – Clindamycin

➢ Differential

- Give 3 non-infectious conditions which may mimic infectious cellulitis.

  - o FMF (familial Mediterranean fever)
    - Erysipelas-like, usually unilateral lesion on low leg / foot

  - o Erythromelalgia
    - Redness of extremities
      - Warm burning
      - Paroxysmal

  - o Sweet syndrome
    - Acute febrile neutrophilic dermatitis
    - Usually affects
      - Middle-aged women
      - Papules / plaques
      - Tender
    - Site
      - Upper extremities
      - Neck
      - Upper trunk

- Give the empiric therapy for purulent cellulitis.

  - o Because of the concern that the causative organism could be CA-MRSA (community-associated methicillin-resistant Staphylococcus aureus), the suggested antibiotic choices would include
    - Trimethroprim-sulfamethoxazole; doxycycline, clindamycin and linezolid

Staphylococcus aureus

➢ Pathophysiology

- o Genes encoding for cytotoxins which
  - Destroy WBC
  - Cause tissue necrosis

➢ Common presentations

- o Purulent SSTIs

- o Pneumonia

➢ Treatment (empiric antibiotics)

- Give the empiric antibodies recommended for MRSA diagnosed in an outpatient (community) or hospital (nosacominal) setting.

  - o In an outpatient setting
    - Trimethoprin-sulfamethoxazole
    - Tetracycline
    - Linezolid
    - Clindamycin
      - Monitor clindamycin resistance in your area of practice, and do not use empirically for MRSA in resistance > 10%
  - o In a hospital setting
    - Linezolid (also covers B-hemolytic streptococci)
    - Vancomycin
    - Ceftaroline
    - Telavancin

SO YOU WANT TO BE AN INFECTIOUS DISEASE EXPERT!

- Give the molecular **mechanism** for the develop of methicillin-resistant Staphylococcus aureus, and explain why ceftaroline is effective against MRSA.

  - o Staphylococcus aureus organism acquire the gene MUC

  - o MUC encodes for the membrane penicillin-binding protein 2a

  - o This penicillin-binding protein 2a in the membrane of S. aureus has a low affinity of β-lactam agents

  - o Ceftaroline is a fifth-generation cephalosporin which has a high affinity for penicillin-binding protein 2, and is thus effective against MRSA.

Abbreviations: CSF, cerebrospinal fluid; UTI, urinary tract infection

---

Internal Medicine: *Infectious disease*
A. B. R. Thomson

Necrotizing Fasciitis

➢ Definition: "necrotizing fasciitis is an SSTI [skin and soft tissue infection] that extends beyond the epidermis, dermis and subcutaneous fat tissue to the fascia and potentially, the underlying muscle."

➢ Types
   o Type I   polymicrobial
   o Type II   monomicrobial

➢ Diagnosis
   o High index of clinical suspicion
   o MRI

A patient with compensated cirrhosis from iron overload presents with hemorrhagic bullae and sepsis after cutting his fat on a sharp stick while swimming in the ocean off Mexico. Necrotizing fasciitis is diagnosed.
- Give the likely causative organism.

   o The likely organism is Vibrio vulnificus, to which the patient is more prone because of the cirrhosis and the excess iron.

➢ Treatment
   o Emergent (MR ~ 50%)
   o Surgical debridement, respected daily, as indicated
   o Empiric antibiotics

- Give the organisms causing type I and type II necrotizing fasciitis, and the recommended empiric antibiotics.

Organisms	Type I (polymicrobial)	Type II (monomicrobial)

	o Staphylococci
	o Streptococci
	o Aerobic gram-negative bacilli
	o Anaerobes
	  – Clostridium
	  – Bacteroides
	  – Peptostreptococcus
		o Streptococcus pyogens
		o St. agalactiae
		o Vibrio vulnificus
		o S. aureus
		o Clostridium perfringens

Internal Medicine: *Infectious disease*
A. B. R. Thomson

- o Necrotizing fasciitis due to Streptococci develop TSS (toxic shock syndrome – please see next subsection) in 50%

  - – Type I
    - ▪ Vancomycin, linezolid, or deptomycin, plus
    - ▪ Piperacillin-tazobactam ("pip-tazo"), or
    - ▪ Metronidazole plus cefepime, or
    - ▪ Meropenem, or imepenem
  - – Type II (monomicrobial, GABHS or clostridium)
    - ▪ Penicillin plus clindamycin

Note: Use of IVIG (IV immune globulin) is controversial, and generally used if TSS has developed, or if there is "a high risk of death" (remember that the overall MR [mortality rate] for necrotizing fasciitis is 30% to 70%)

MCQ Alert

There are unique presentations for V. vulnificus that makes it a "must" for a multiple choice question (MCQ).

- o Gram-negative rod

- o Common in coastal waters of Mexico
  - - Break in skin, swimming

- o High risk for
  - - Immunocompromised
  - - Hemosiderosis / hemochromatosis

- o Associated pain is severe and out of proportion to skin changes

---

Toxic Shock Syndrome (TSS)

- ➢ Causes / associations
  - o Toxin-producing Staphylococcus and Streptococci
  - o May be associated with necrotizing fasciitis

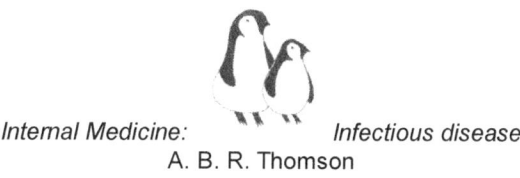

- Give 10 conditions with the development of toxic shock syndrome (TSS).
    - Menstruation, especially with use of tampons
    - Infections
        - Surgery / blunt trauma
        - Childbirth
        - Nose
            - Sinus infection with nose packing
        - Skin
        - Bone
        - Pnemonia
        - Influenza ⎫
        - Varicella ⎭ for TSS from Streptococcus
    - Medication
        - NSAIDs (for TSS from Streptococcus)
    - Injections
        - IVDU (IV drug use)
    - Localizing signs are not necessarily present

- ➤ Clinical
    - Diagnostic criteria have been established for TSS, depending upon whether the causative organism is Staphylococcal (S. pyogens or B-hemolytic Streptococcus [GABHS])

- ➤ Prophylaxis (for secondary transmission of GABHS - TSS)
    - Penicillin-based prophylaxis
    - Contact isolation until 24 h after first day of empiric antibiotics completed in index patient
        - Close contacts
        - Others
            - household contacts
            - Diabetics
            - CV disease
            - Cancer
            - IVDU
            - Infection
                - HIV
                - Varicella
            - Users of corticosteroids

Internal Medicine: *Infectious disease*
A. B. R. Thomson

Viral infections

- **Epstein Barr Virus (EBV)**

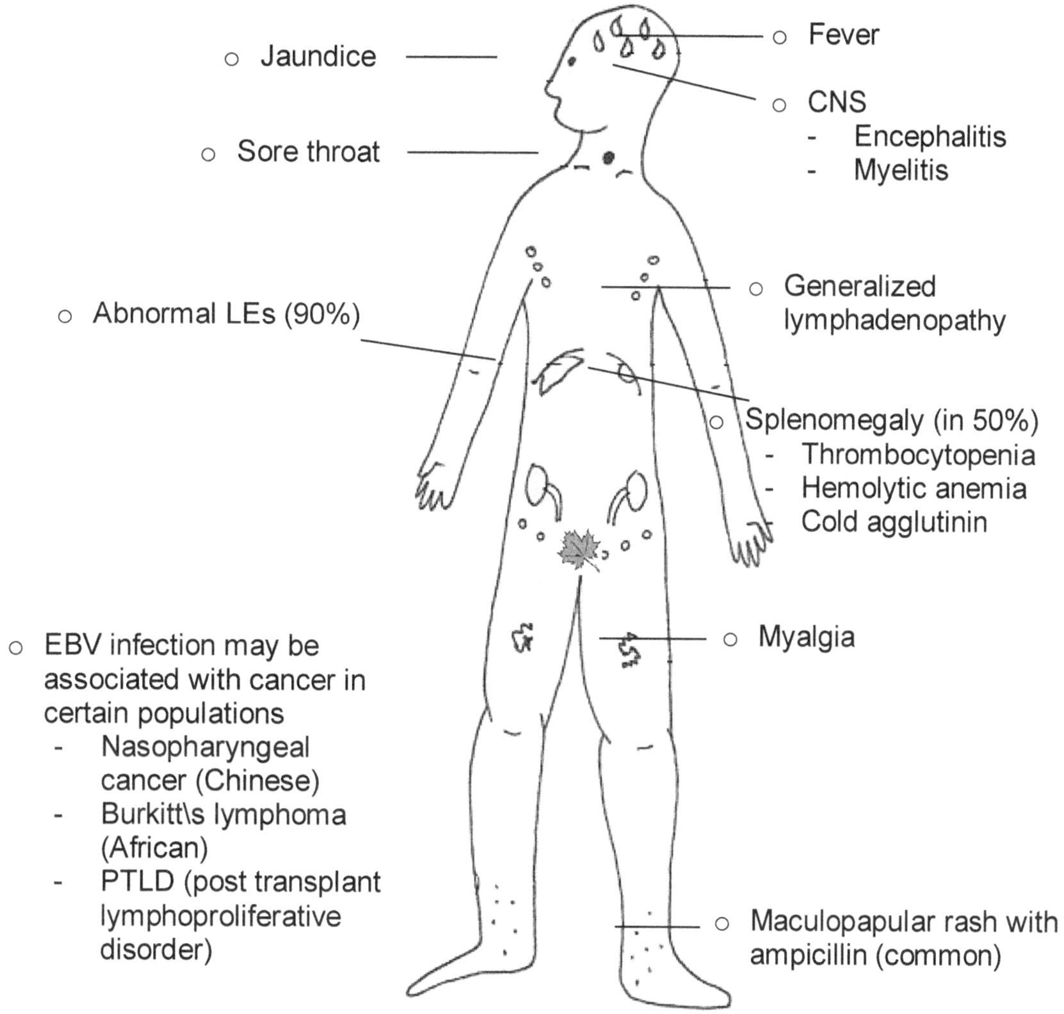

  - Jaundice ——————
  - Sore throat ——————————
  - Abnormal LEs (90%)

  - o Fever
  - o CNS
    - Encephalitis
    - Myelitis
  - o Generalized lymphadenopathy
  - o Splenomegaly (in 50%)
    - Thrombocytopenia
    - Hemolytic anemia
    - Cold agglutinin
  - o Myalgia
  - o Maculopapular rash with ampicillin (common)

  - o EBV infection may be associated with cancer in certain populations
    - Nasopharyngeal cancer (Chinese)
    - Burkitt\s lymphoma (African)
    - PTLD (post transplant lymphoproliferative disorder)

Adapted from: Davey P. *Wiley-Blackwell* 2006, page 298.

- ➢ Clinical
  - o EBV infection is usually associated with infectious mononucleosis syndrome (IMS) (flu-like illness, fever, posterior cervical lymphoadenopathy, aplenomegaly, sore throat, measles-like rash after ampicillin, atypical peripheral blood lymphocytes and positive serology).
  - o Some patients may have atypical presentations.

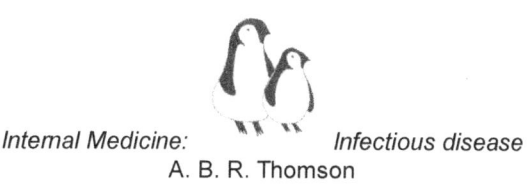

Internal Medicine: *Infectious disease*
A. B. R. Thomson

- Give 4 presentations of EBV infection other than the typical IMS or EBV-associated malignancies.

  - CNS   – Aseptic meningitis
    -               – Aseptic encephalitis

  - Liver   – Hepatitis

  - Blood   – Hemolytic anemia
    -               – Thrombocytopenia

- Give 3 viruses which are associated with IMS (infectious mononucleosis syndrome)

  - EBV

  - CMV

  - HIV

- Complications

- Give 4 **malignant or premalignant conditions** associated with EBV

  - Lymphoma   – B-cell
    -               – T-cell
    -               – Hodgkin
    -               – PTLD (post-transplantation lymphoproliferative disorder)

  - Leukoplakia, oral hairy   – Painless, white, corrugated plaques on edge of tongue

  - Nasopharyngeal carcinoma

- Diagnosis

- Give the serological tests for present and past EBV infection.

		EBV Infection	
		Present acute primary	Past
o	Viral capsid antigen IgM	↑	0
o	Early antigen IgE	↑	0
o	Epstein-Barr nuclear antigen-1 IgE	↓ / 0	↑

Note; VCA (viral capsid antigen) IgG is increased in both, thus does not help to distinguish between present and past EBV infection

➢ Treatment

  o Conservative

  o No anti-viral drugs

  o Corticosteroids for severe
    – Lung disease
    – Hemolytic anemia

- **Varicella-Zoster Virus (VZV) Infections**

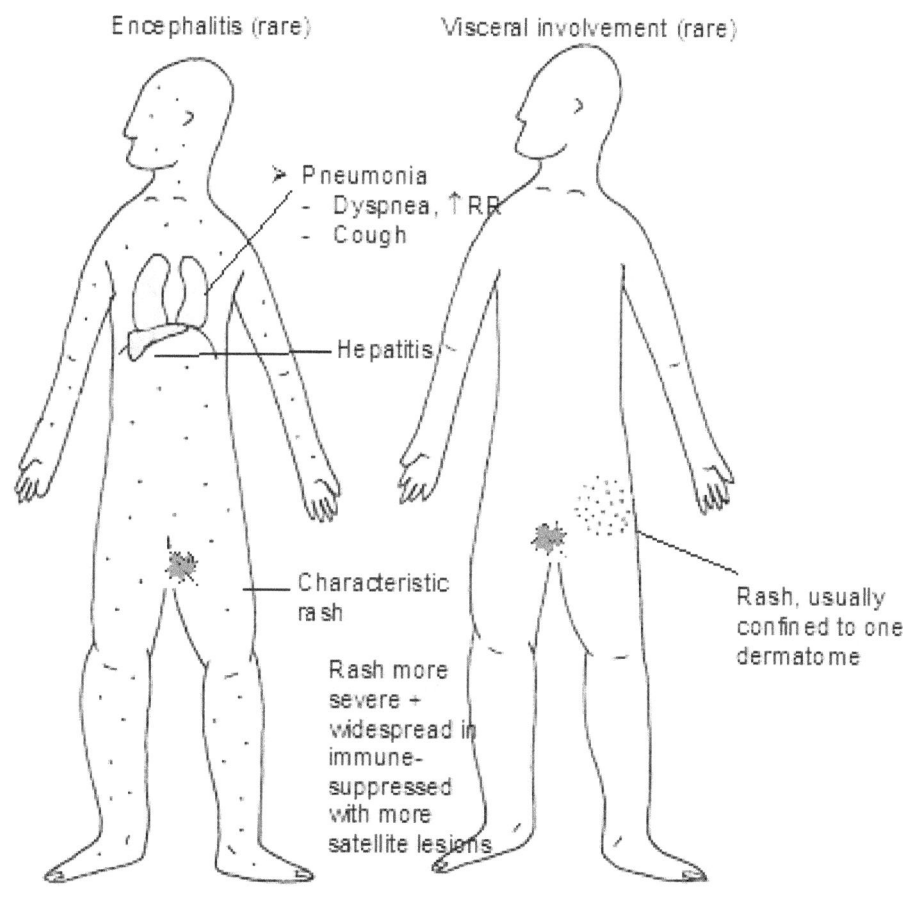

Encephalitis (rare)   Visceral involvement (rare)

➢ Pneumonia
  – Dyspnea, ↑RR
  – Cough

Hepatitis

Characteristic
rash

Rash more
severe +
widespread in
immune-
suppressed
with more
satellite lesions

Rash, usually
confined to one
dermatome

1° infection (chickenpox)   Reactivation (Zoster)

Adapted from: Davey P. *Wiley-Blackwell* 2006, page 298.
- **Chickenpox**   o Varicella vaccine

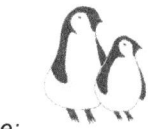

Internal Medicine: *Infectious disease*
A. B. R. Thomson

- o VZIB (varicella zoster immune globulin)
- o VariZIG (varicella zoster immune globulin) product

- **Shingles**
  - o Vaccine for > age 60 yr
  - o Antivirals
    - – Acyclovir
    - – Valacyclovir
    - – Famciclovir

- **Cytomegalovirus (CMV)**

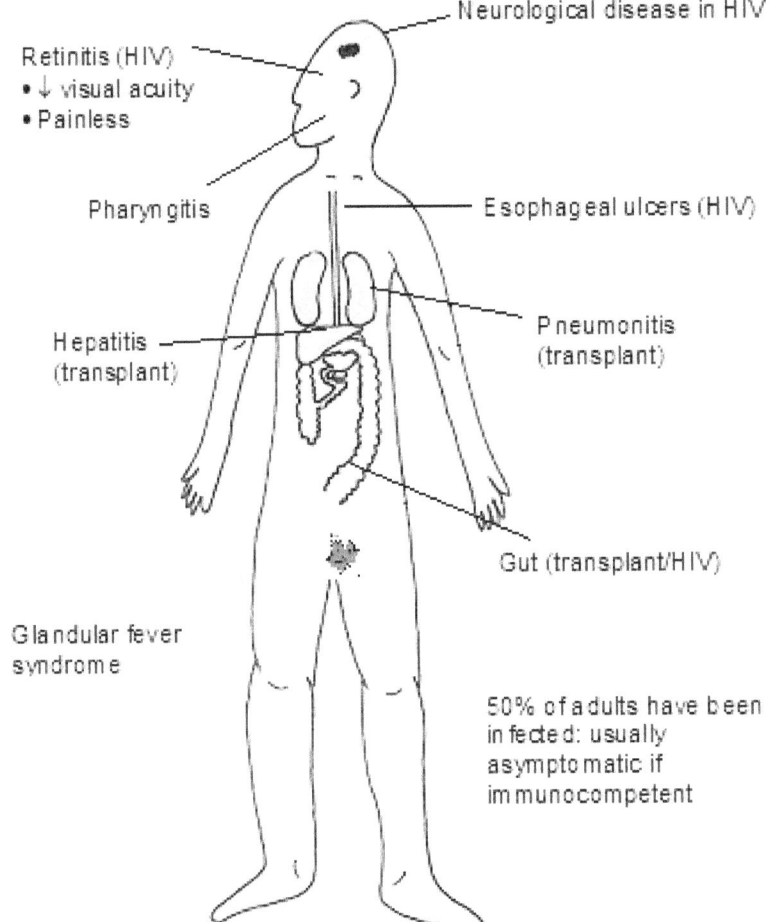

Adapted from: Davey P. *Wiley-Blackwell* 2006, page 298.

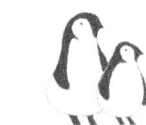

- Give the treatment of choice to be given within 4 days (96 hr) to the pregnant or immunocompromised person who has been exposed to varicella.

    o VariZIG immune globulin, or

    o Immune globulin IV

    o Do not give varicella vaccine
      - Live virus is usually contraindicated in immunosuppressed patient

VIRAL HEMORRHAGIC FEVERS (VHF)

➢ Causes / associations
  o RNA viruses, including Yellow fever, Dengue fever, Embola hemorrhagic fever

  o Potential of per-to-person transmission

➢ Clinical

  o Procedures widespread vascular damage e.g.
    - Petechial hemorrhages
    - Conjunctival injection
    - Hypotension

➢ Diagnosis (specialized diagnosis)

  o Detect viral protein antigens

  o IgM antibodies

  o PCR

  o Culture

➢ Treatment

  o Supportive care

Ebola

➢ Microbiology
  o Ebola virus (EV) is a filoviridae with a lipid envelop, genome base 10 kb, and icosahedral-shaped organism causing a febrile illness in the setting of a multi-system disease. Some of the filamentous virions fuse end-to-end, resulting in athe apprearance of a "bowel of spaghetti".

Internal Medicine: *Infectious disease*
A. B. R. Thomson

- o The may survive for weeks at room temperature in dry blood.
- o The Ebola virus is a biosafety level 4 pathogen because of its high (~50%) mortality rate.

➢ Clinical

- o Infection in the mononuclear phagocytic system leads to widespread cellular necrosis including cerebral necrosis of glial with infarction, interstitial pneumonitis, hepatitis, a skin rash and bleeding from any mucosal surface, such as the GI tract.
- o The role of possible aerosol infectivity is controversial.

➢ Laboratory

- o Viremia is detected by ELISA and RT-PCR is commonly positive, with IgG and IgM autoantibodies developing in survivors.

➢ Treatment

- o There is no preventive vaccine, or proven anti-viral drug.
- o Pharmaceuticals studied in non-human primates, such as an adenovirus-vectored glycoprotein gene, are being rushed to human use in the recent West African epidemic.
- o Treatment is confined to isolation, hydration, nutrition, and public health measures to prevent epidemicization.

- For 10 of the following "**Buzzwords**", give the likely pathogen on infection.

Buzzwords used in MCQ	Implication
o Atypical lymphocytes, heterophile antibody positive	– EBV
o Bell palsy syndrome	– HSV
o Bulbar palsy plus flaccid paralysis, or "Five D's"	– Botulism
o Conjunctival suffusion	– Leptospira interogans
o Deep bone culture	– Osteomyelitis
o Jarisch-Herxheimer reaction	– T-pallidum (syphilis)

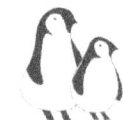

Internal Medicine: *Infectious disease*
A. B. R. Thomson

Buzzwords used in MCQ	Implication
○ Non-tender, red macules on palms and soles	– Infectious endocarditis (Janeway lesion)
○ Oral hairy leukoplakia	– HIV
○ Painless, pruritic papule with black eschar, plus wide mediastinum on chest x-ray	– Anthrax
○ Papules and vesicles all at the same stage, beginning in the face	– Smallpox
○ PML (progressive multifocal [eukoencephalopathy]	– Polymavirus JC
○ Pneumothorax in HIV infected person	– Pneumocystis jiovecci
○ Whitlow	– HSV
○ West Africa, world-wide epidemic	– Ebola virus

TICK-BORNE DISEASE

- ○ Lyme disease
- ○ Babesiosis
- ○ Southern-Tick-Associated Rash Illness (STARI)
- ○ Ehrlichiosis and Anaplasmosis
- ○ Rocky Mountain Spotted Fever (RMSF)

- Give 3 tick-borne pathogens treated with doxycycline.

- ○ Lyme diseaseergdorferi
  - – Borrelia b
- ○ Human granulocytic anaplasmosis
  - – Anaplasma phagocytophilum
- ○ Rocky Mountain spotted fever (RMSF)
  - – Rickettsia rickettsii

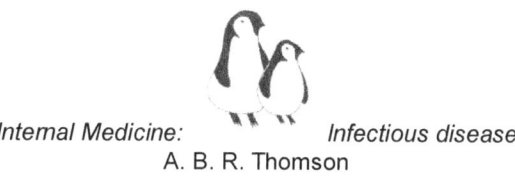

Internal Medicine: *Infectious disease*
A. B. R. Thomson

Lyme Disease

➤ Causes / associations

    o Vector deer tick
- – Ixodes scapularis

    o Causative spirochete

    o Note
- – May be associated with co-infection with Babesia micoti, causing Babesiosis

➤ Clinical

               1-2 wk

Tick attachment ⟶ Early localized (EM, erythema migrans) ⟶

Spirochetemia
⟶ Early disseminated ⟶ Late

    o When a patient presents with a skin rash from the appropriate endemic area of Lyme disease, only about half will remember tick attachment, and the initial skin lesion may be EM (erythema migrans). Because it is important to treat this tick-borne disease early to prevent later serious complications, it is important to recognize early localized Lyme disease.

• Give a description of the typical **erythema migrans** (EM) of Lyme disease.

    o An expansile, target-like skin lesion, often associated with a tick bite or attachment causing Lyme disease or Southern tick-associated rash illness.

    o Centre
- – Clear (looks like a "bulls-eye")
- – May become necrotic or vesicular

    o Edges
- – May become confluent macule

    o Associated cellulitis

    o EM may spread to skin sites distant from the initial attachment

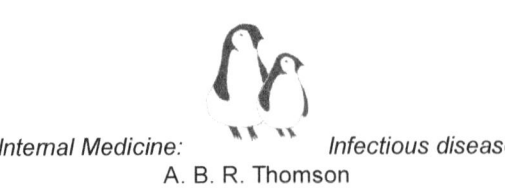

- Give the name of the infectious cause of EM which may mimic Lyme disease but occurs in the Southern USA.

    o STARI (Southern tick-associated rash illness)

➤ Early-disseminated disease

    o Incubation period, 3 to 6 wk

    o Febrile illness, with lymphadenopathy

    o Heart
      – Myocarditis (5%)
      – Heart block

    o CNS
      – CN palsy, unilateral or bilateral
      – Aseptic meningitis
      – Radiculopathy

➤ Late-stage disease (60%)

    o Incubation period, months to years

    o Joints   – Migratory, mono- or oligoarticular arthritis
                      – Knee induced in 85%
                      – Remission and recurrences years later

    o CNS   – Encephalopathy
                      – Encephalitis

➤ Post-Lyme Disease Syndrome

    o "…….. patients with confirmed Lyme disease, based on clinical and laboratory criteria, who have persistent constitutional symptoms despite appropriate antibiotic treatment"

    o Supportive treatment only

    o Testing

      – Do not test an asymptomatic person after a tick bite
      – "……. restricted primarily to patients with clinically suggestive signs or symptoms (other than erythema migrans) who reside in or have travelled to an endemic area" (MKSAP 16, Infectious disease 2012, page 26)

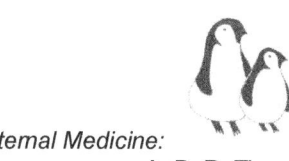

➤ Diagnosis

 o Blood

  – Positive or equivocal ELISA test for antibody to B. burgdorferi, followed by

  – Confirmatory Western blotting

  – If only 1 more of symptoms / signs (other than EM) IgM antibody

  – The finding of B. burgdorferi antibodies in patients who have non-specific symptoms of fatigue or myalgia or who are unlikely to have been exposed to a water tick likely represents a false-positive test result for Lyme disease, be treated.

Lies about Lyme Disease

 o "Early Lyme disease is diagnosed with serology testing."

  – "No": serology testing may be negative for early Lyme disease

  – The earlier sign of Lyme disease is "erythema migrans", large red rings on the skin.

 o Be satisfied that "treatment for Lyme disease is satisfactory when the titer of antibody falls."

  – "No": serology testing is not a reliable gauge for adequacy of treatment.

 o "The treatment of choice for Borrelia burdorferi infection is amoxicillin."

  – Not quite a "lie"

▪ Empiric treatment	– Amoxicillin
	– Cefuroxime
	– Doxycycline
▪ Lyme-associated carditis or CNS disease	– Ceftriaxone
▪ Arthritis or facial palsy	– Doxycycline

 o "The treatment of Lyme disease in pregnancy is – doxycycline" ??? No-No-No!

  – "lie, **BIG BAD LIE**": doxycycline must **not** be given in pregnancy

---

Internal Medicine: *Infectious disease*
A. B. R. Thomson

➢ Treatment

• Give the treatment of the patient with Lyme disease, caused Borrelia burgdorferi, who develops bradycardia (Lyme myocarditis).

- o 1ˢᵗ degree HB (heart block), asymptomatic — Outpatient cefuroxime, or doxycycline po
- o 2ⁿᵈ or 3ʳᵈ degree HB — Impatient monitoring
  - IV ceftriaxone

• Give the empiric treatment of erythema migrans,

- o It is not necessary to distinguish between which tick-borne infection is causing the EM.
- o Begin treatment of the EM with doxycycline

Babesiosis

➢ Causes / associations
- o Directly, from tick-borne protozoal infection with Babesia microti
- o Transfusion with infected blood

➢ Clinical course
- o Organism relicates in RBCs, and may be
  - Asymptomatic, or progress to
  - Blood
    - Hemolysis
    - DIC
  - Kidney
  - Heart
    - HF
  - Multi-organ failure

Abbreviations: AKI, acute kidney injury; DIC, disseminated intravascular coagulation; HF, heart failure

➢ Diagnosis
- o PCR of blood for B. microti
- o RBC thin
  - Ring forms of B. microti in RBCs
  - Do not confuse with Malaria falciparum
- o For symptoms, or asymptomatic parasitemia > 3 mon

➤ Treatment
  o Mild
    – Atovaquone plus azithromycin or quinine and clindamycin
  o Sever
    – Atovaquone plus quinine and clindamycin
    – Exchange transfusion

Southern Tick-Associated Rash Illness (STARI)

  o Southern USA
  o EM in early stage
  o Vector in the tick Ambylomma americanum; causative agent unknown
  o Does not progress
  o Treat with doxycycline 100 mg bid po for 1 to 2 wk (again, do **not** use in pregnancy).

Ehrlichiosis and Anaplasmosis

➤ Cause / associations
  o Tick-borne diseases
  o HME
    – Human granulocyte Ehrlichiosis
      ▪ Lone star tick SE, SC, mid-Atlantic USA
  o HGA
    – Human granulocyte anaplasmosis
      ▪ Deer tick NE, NC USA

➤ Clinical
  o Febrile illness
  o Usually no skin, but when present
    – Maculopapular
    – Petechial
  o Meningoencephalitis in < 20%

➤ Laboratory
  o Blood
    – Abnormal Les (liver enzymes)
    – Lymphopenia, thrombocytopenia
    – Buffy coat, clusters of bacteria in WBCs
  o CSF
    – Pleocytosis, lymphocytic
    – ↑ protein

➤ Treatment
  o Doxycycline 100 mg bid po for 7 to 14 days

(caution: do **not** use in pregnancy)
- o Treat early to ↓ MR (mortality rate)

Rocky Mountain Spotted Fever (RMSF)

- ➢ Causes / associations
  - o Tick-borne rickettsial disease
  - o Rickettsia Rickettsii

- ➢ Clinical
  - o Fever
  - o GI symptoms
  - o Skin rash
    - – early 15%
    - – Late 90%
    - – Macules
    - – No blanching
    - – Wrists, ankles → petechial everywhere except on the face

- ➢ Laboratory
  - o Abnormal Les (liver enzymes)
  - o Thrombocytopenia
  - o No lymphopenia or leukopenia (as in HME or HGA)
  - o Serological testing
    - – Positive, or
    - – Seroconversion on convalescent serum
  - o Skin biopsy
    - – Positive for R. rickettsia

- ➢ Treatment
  - o Doxycycline 100 mg po for 1-2 wk

"Use diagnostic imaging to guide your clinical impression, not to make the diagnosis."

Dr. Joel Hurwitz

Internal Medicine: *Infectious disease*
A. B. R. Thomson

HIV / AIDS

➢ Definition
- o CD4 count < 200 / mL
- o AIDS-indicating opportunistic
  - – Infections
  - – Malignancies

➢ Diagnosis
- o HIV
  - – Two-stage serological testing (may be negative in AS [acute retroviral infection])
  - – Repeat testing of positive EIA (enzyme immunoassay) by Western blotting
  - – Performance characteristics
    - ▪ Sensitivity 99.5%
    - ▪ Specificity 99.99%
  - – When EIA positive but Western blot negative
    - ▪ False-positive EIA
  - – Indeterminate Western blot on repeat testing cross-reacting antibody due to infection
  - – Quantitative RNA-PCR (polymerase chain reaction)

➢ Clinical

One of the major indications for HAART / ART therapy in the patient with HIV infection is history of an AIDS-defining illness (opportunistic infection or malignancy).

- Give 15 **AIDs-defining illnesses**.

➢ Site
- o CNS
  - – HIV
  - – Encephalopathy
  - – Toxoplasmosis
  - – Lymphoma (primary)
  - – Progressive multiple leukoencephalopathy)
- o Eye
  - – CMV retinitis
- o Lung
  - – Candidiasis
  - – HSV
  - – Bronchitis / pneumonitis
  - – Lymphoid interstitial pneumonia
  - – Recurrent bacterial pneumonia

- GI
  - Candidiasis of esophagus
  - HSV of esophagus
  - HIV wasting syndrome
  - Chronic
    - Cyptosporidiosis
    - Isosoporiasis

- GU
  - Cervical cancer (invasive)

➢ Organism
- Extrapulmonary
  - Coccidiodomycosis
  - Cryptococcosis
  - Histoplasmosis

➢ Tumors
- Kaposi sarcoma

- Lymphoma
  - Burkitt
  - Immunoblastic

- Mycobacterium tuberculosis

- Extrapulmonary
  - MAC (Mycobacterium avium complex)
  - MK (Mycobacterium kansasii)

- Pneumocytis jirovecii

- Salmonella bacteremia, recurrent

- CMV infection other than LSLN (liver, spleen, lymph nodes)

Adapted from: MKSAP 16, Infectious disease 2012, Table 54, page 92.

SO YOU WANT TO BE AN ID CONSULTANT!

- In the context of a person with HIV/AIDs, what is **eosinophilic folliculitis**?
  - An infection of hair follicles, typically papular, pruritic and seen in HIV-infected persons

Clinical Alert

Primary prophylaxis is recommended in HIV / AIDS when the CD4 count is < 200 / μL for Pneumocystis jirocecii, < 100 / ml and positive serology for toxoplasmosis, < 50 μL for MAC (mycobacterium avium complex), and tuberculin skin test (TST) > 5 mm or positive IGRA (interferon γ release assay) for tuberculosis.

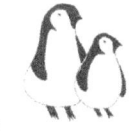

- Give the precaution necessary before therapy with TMP / SMX, azithromycin, and INH (isoniazid).

    o Exclude acute infection with MAC (blood cultures) on TB to ↓ development of resistance and use of inadequate drug doses

---

Clinical Gem

- Beware the "company" that diseases keep.

In the patient with oral hairy leukoplakia, and an EBV infection, give the other viral infection which must be excluded.

    o Oral hairy leukoplakia is very highly suggestive of an infection with HIV

- Give the **criteria for screening** for HIV infection.

    o The answer may vary by country policy
    o For USA, the CDC (Centres for Disease Control and Preventions" ………recommend HIV screening for all persons between the age of 13 and 64 years at least once and--- these with risk factors [should] undergo annual testing". (MKSAP 16, Infectious disease 2012, page 181)

➢ Prophylaxis
    o Pre-exposure emtricitabine / tenofovir
        – HIV (-ive) person having sexual activity with HIV (+ive) person
    o Post-exposure early use of drugs after exposure
        – Occupational, and possibly sexual
    o Perinatal screening
        – ART (antiretroviral therapy) to ↓ risk of transmission to fetus

➢ Treatment
- Give the current guidelines for anti-retroviral (ART, HAART) treatment of HIV infection.
    o Symptoms of HIV infection (please see above)
    o CD4 ≤ 500 /μL
    o AIDS-deficiency illness (opportunistic infection or malignancy)
    o HIV-nephropathy

- o Co-infection, HBV / HCV
- o Pregnancy and HIV infection (HAART reduces HIV transmission from 25% → 2%

Treatment combination regimens

- o Standard preferred starting regimen (maybe modified by sensitivity testing)
  - 2 nucleodise RTIs (tenofovir plus emtricitabine), plus
  - 1 non-nucleoside RTI (efavirenz), or
  - 1 potease inhibitor
  - Atazanavir or darunavir, plus
  - Small dose of ritonavir
  - Other regimens used in pregnancy: lamivudine and zidovydine, plus
  - Lopinavir or ritonavir (protease inhibitors)

Abbreviation: RTI, reverse transcriptase inhibitor

- • Give adverse effects / complications of **HAART therapy**.

  - o HAART (antiviral therapy with highly active antiviral therapy) is associated with

o Metabolic disorders	–	Lipids
		▪ ↓ total HDL, LDH cholesterol concentrations
		▪ ↑ serum triglyceride
	–	Lipodystrophy
	–	Insulin resistance
		▪ ↑ faslting glucose
		▪ ↑ Hg A1C
	–	Metabolic lactic acidosis
o Bone	–	↑ osteopenia
	–	↑ osteoporosis
o Kidney	–	HIV nephropathy
o Liver	–	↑ risk of co-infection with HBV / HCV
	–	↑ risk of progression to cirrhosis (HIV plus HCV)
o CVS	–	↑ atherosclerosis
	–	↑ cardiac deaths
o IRIS (immune reconstitution inflammatory syndrome)	–	Reconstitution of the immune system which occurs weeks to months after starting HAART results in a marked inflammatory response, especially against TB and fungal infections

o Opportunistic Infections

CD4 cell count per µL	Organism / Infection
> 200	Candidiasis
< 200	Pneumocystis jirovecii
< 100	Cryptococcus
< 50	Toxoplasma gondii CMV MAC (Mycobacterium avium) TB Poxvirus Molluscum contagiosum Bortonella bacillary angiomatosis HHV-8 Kaposi sarcoma caused by human herpes virus

CASE CHALLENGE

A pregnant woman who has no-HIV-associated symptoms form her infection has a normal CD4 count, and her viral load is low. From her reading, she does not require HAART, and she is concerned about the teratogenicity of the HAART drugs such as efaviranz.

- Give your advice about the treatment of an HIV infection during **pregnancy**.
  - o It is time that there are criteria to follow before stating HAART for an HIV infection
  - o However, all HIV-infected pregnant woman should be treated to prevent transmission of HIV to the fetus (25% → 2%)
  - o While efavirenz is contraindicated in pregnancy, other regimens are safe.
  - o She reads treatment with a regimen such as lamivudine plus zidovudine and lopinavir-ritonavir

- In the patient with suboptimally controlled HIV RNA viral loads despite usually appropriate HAART therapy, give the reason why **resistance testing** is performed while the patient remains on HAART.
  - o A drug "holiday" (stopping HAART) would only lead to ↑ HIV load
  - o "resistance testing done while the patient is not receiving [HAART] therapy may be unreliable without the selective pressure of the medications to maintain the presence of mutations in the predominant [resistant] viral population" (MKSAP 16, Infectious disease 2012, page 170)

ACUTE RETROVIRAL SYNDROME (ARS)

- o Fibrile illness 2-4 wk after exposure
- o High viral loads due to early lack of immune response
- o HIV testing still negative in the window interval, until seroconversion occurs
- o Not yet clear whether ART (antiviral therapy) beneficial for ARS

CHRONIC HIV INFECTION

- o HIV infects CD4 T-lymphocytes which replicate, integrate into genome of host cells, and cause immune compromise
- o Non-opportunistic infections become more
    - – Common
    - – Severe
    - – Prolonged
- o Examples include

– Mouth	▪	HSV (herpes simplex virus) infection
– Lung	▪	Pneumococcal pneumonia
– GU	▪	Vaginal candidiasis recurrent / refractory
	▪	HZV (herpes zoster infection)
	▪	Genital HSV infection

- • Give 10 common clinical features of chronic HIV infection

- ➢ Clinical
    - o Systemic
        - – Fever
        - – Night sweats
        - – Fatigue
        - – ↓ weight
    - o Mouth
        - – Aphthous ulcers
        - – Hairy leukoplakia
        - – Gingivitis
        - – Periodontitis
    - o Skin
        - – Seborrhic dermatitis
        - – Psoriasis
        - – Tinea
        - – Onychomycosis

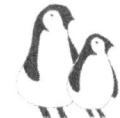

- o GI   – Diarrhea
- o GU   – Nephropathy
- o CNS / PNS   – Peripheral neuropathy
- o Blood   – Cytopenia

Adapted from MKSAP 16, Infectious disease 2012, Table 50, page 87.

SEXUALLY TRANSMITTED DISEASES

- For an excellent background for how to take a directed history for STD (sexually transmitted disease), see: Jugovic PJ, et al. *Saunders/ Elsevier* 2004, pages 89 and 90.

Useful background: Sexually transmitted pathogens and the disease which each causes.
- o Chlamydia trachomatis (chlamydia)
- o Neisseria gonorrhoeae (gonorrhea)
- o   Herpes simplex virus (HSV; herpes)
- o Hepatitis B and C (hepatitis)
- o Human Immunodeficiency Virus (HIV/AIDS)
- o Trepomena pallidum (syphilis)
- o Human papilloma virus (genital warts)

Source: Jugovic PJ, et al. *Saunders/ Elsevier* 2004, page 90.

- o Cervicitis, urethritis   – Chlamdia trachomatis
  Proctitis, Eididymitis   – Neissera gonorrhoeae
- o Epididymitis
- o Genital ulcers   – HSV infection
                                    – Syphilis
                                    – Chancroid
                                    – Lymphogranuloma venereum
- o Genital warts   – Condylomata acuminanta (HPV)

- Give the **complications** of sexually transmitted diseases **in women.**
  - Acute salpingitis
  - Pelvic inflammatory disease
  - Infertility
  - Ectopic pregnancies
  - Arthritis
  - Conjunctivitis
  - Urethritis
  - Fitz-Hugh-Curtis syndrome GC/ (chlamydial infection of the liver capsule)

Source: Jugovic PJ, et al. *Saunders/ Elsevier* 2004, pages 90 and 91.

Chlamydia trachomatis

➢ Demography	o < 25 yr

	o Sex
	   – Unprotected
	   – Multiple partners
	   – New partners

➢ Clinical	o Cervicitis
	o Urethritis
	o Proctitis
➢ Complications in women	o Infertility
	o PID (pelvic inflammatory disease)
	o Ectopic pregnancy

➢ Diagnosis	o Discharge swab / urine
	   – Culture
	   – NAA (nucleic acid amplification) testing

	o Screen
	   – Sexually active women ≤ 25 yr
	   – Other high risk factors

	o Check sexual partners
	   – From time of symptom
	      ▪ All sex partners in last 60 days
	      ▪ Last sex partner if > 60 days

➢ Treatment
- o Ceftriaxone, 250 mg IM, one dose, plus
- o Azothromycin, 1 g po, one dose, or
- o Cefixime, 400 mg po, one dose, plus
- o Doxycycline 100 mg po bid for 7 days

Note: High rate of co-infection with N. gonorrhoeae

Pelvic Inflammatory Disease (PID)

➢ Definition
- o A polymicrobial infection (usually C. trachomatis plus N. gonorrhoeae) arising from infection ascending from the cervix, to cause
  - – Endometritis
  - – Salpingitis (or salpingitis plus endometritis)
  - – Tubo-ovarian abscess
  - – Scarring of fallopian tube (infertility)

➢ Diagnosis
- o High index of suspicion of sexually active young women, especially with fever, ceviates (discharge), tenderness of uterus and adenexia

➢ Treatment
- o Mostly as outpatients, unless PID is complicated
  - – Pregnant
  - – Proven / suspected tubo-ovarian abscess
  - – Failure of outpatient therapy
  - – Systemic toxicity
  - – Possible surgical emergency
- o po / IM
  - – Ceftriaxone, 250 mg, one dose, plus
  - – Doxycycline, 100 mg, po bid for 14 days, plus / -
  - – Metronidazole, 500 mg po bid for 14 days
- o IV
  - – Cefotetan, 2 g q 12 h, or
  - – Cefoxitin, 2 g q 6 h, plus
  - – Doxycycline, 100 mg IV q 12 h

Internal Medicine: *Infectious disease*
A. B. R. Thomson

- Give the recommended antibiotic therapy, which will cover the likely causes of the polymicorbial infection in the patient with cervicitis with or without PID.
  - Without PID
    - Ceftriaxone IM, XI, plus azithromycin PO
  - With PID
    - Neisseria gonorrheae
    - Chlamydia trachomatis
    - Aerobes
    - Anaerobes
  - Antibiotic combinations

No systemic toxicity ceftriaxone IM IX, plus doxycycline PO for 14 days systemic toxicity IM clindamycin

Note: Men who have had sexual contact with a woman with PID need to be evaluated and treated for infection with the organisms noted above.

Epididymitis

➢ Demography	○ < 35 yr	
	– C. trachomatis or N. gonorrhoeae	
	○ Older man ± BPN (benign prostatic hypertrophy)	
	– Enteric gram-negative organisms	
	○ MSM (men who have sex with men, "insertive" partner in anal intercourse)	
	– Enterobacteriaceae	
➢ Clinical	○ Unilateral pain / tenderness in epididymis and testis	
	○ Enlarge / tender spermatic cord	
	○ Urine	
	– WBC ≥ 10 / hpf	
	– Positive dipstick leukocyte esterase	
	○ Note	
	– Differentiate from testicular torsion	
➢ Treatment	○ Ceftriaxone, 250 mg IM, one dose. plus	
	○ Doxycycline, 100 mg bid for 10 days	

Note: With regards to treatment of ceviates, urethritis, PID, epididymitis, please refer to standard medical textbooks or to reviews such as MKSAP 16, Infectious disease 2012, Table 26, page 45.

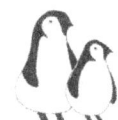

Genital Ulcers

➢ Clinical

    o HSV-1 primary infection
- Skin
  - Vesicles → pustules → ulcers on red base / linear ulcers
- GU
  - Women cervicitis
  - Women and men urethrritis
- Nodes
  - Inguinal lymphadenopathy, tender

    o HSV-2
- Recurrent genital and perianal ulcers
- Subclinical viral shedding is common, with transmission genital ulcers less common

➢ Diagnosis

    o Serological testing

    o Culture

    o NAA tests, e.g. PCR

➢ Treatment

    o Primary infection (usually HSV-1)

    o Recurrent infection, including continued suppressive therapy for > 6 recurrences per year

Please see standard testbook or recent review such as UptoDate or MKSAP 16, Infectious disease 2012, Table 27, page 46

Syphilis

The treatment of syphilis is based on the stage.

- Give the **stages of syphilis** infection.

    o Primary
- Single or multiple round indurated painless chancre with raised border appearing in area of sexual contact
- Genital lesion may be associated with non-tender lymphadenopathy

Internal Medicine: *Infectious disease*
A. B. R. Thomson

- o Secondary
  - Non-pruritic macular, popular or pustular rash on palms and soles
  - An mucosal surface
    - Silvery erosions with red border
- o Tertiary
  - Involvement of CNS (meningovascular, parenchyma), eye, CVS (aortitis)

- Give the difference between early and late latent syphilis.
  - o Asymptomatic (latent), plus serology positive
    - ≤ 1 yr early
    - > 1 yr late / latent, aka syphilis of unknown origin

➢ Treatment
  - o Primary, secondary, early latent
    - Benzathine penicillin G, 2.4 million units IM, one dose, or
    - Doxycycline, 100 mg po bid for 14 days

  - o Late latent
    - Benzathine penicillin G, 3-4 milllion units IM qw for 3 wk, or
    - Doxycycline, 100 mg po bid for 28 days

  - o Neurosyphilis
    - Aqueous crystaliine peniclillin G, 3-4 million units IV q 4 h for 10-14 days, or
    - 18-24 million units IV continuous infusion, per day for 10-14 days

Please see a standard textbook or recent review UptoDate or MKSAP 16, Infectious disease 2012, Table 28, page 47.

CLINICAL CHALLENGE

- In the context of the antibiotic treatment of syphilis, give the clinical feature of the **Jarish Herxheimer reaction**.

  - o The antibiotic kills the syphilitic spirochetes, within 2 hr releasing an endofoxin.

  - o The endotoxin causes fever myalgia headache, skin rash and hypotension.

  - o The patient is treated sytomatically, and the antibiotic is continued if necessary.

  - o Curiously, the Jarish-Herxheimer reaction is more common during pregnancy.

Chancroid

➤	Causes / associations	○ C. trachomatis
➤	Clinical	○ Papule / perianal painless ulcers
		○ Proctocolitis
		○ Painful unilateral inguinal lymphadenopathy – Suppuration, drainage
➤	Diagnosis	○ NAA testing, including PCR
➤	Treatment	○ Doxycycline, 100 mg po bid for 21 day, or
		○ Erythromycin, 500 mg qid for 21 day

The Three Musketeers plus d'Artagnan

For a mucopurulent urethral discharge in a male, cervicitis in a female,

- Give the 4 most likely pathogens which may be part of a co-infection.
  - Neisseria gonorrhoeae
  - Chlamydia
  - HIV
  - Syphilis

- Give the 4 most likely pathogens for genital ulcers.

  - Chancroid (Haemophilus ducreyi)
  - HSV (Herpes simplex virus 1 or 2)
  - LGV (lymphogranuloma venereum; C. trachomatis)
  - Syphilis (T. palladium)

Vaginitis

- Give the commonest causes of vaginitis.

  - Infectious
    - Candidiasis
    - N. gonorrhoeae
    - Chlamydia trachomatis

  - Non-infectious
    - Coitus
    - Allergic reaction to substance to substances placed in vagina
    - Post-menopausal atrophy

- Give conditions associated with HSV infection.
  - Genital herpes
  - HIV (HSV → ↑ transmission rate of HIV)
  - Benign recurrent lymphocytic meningitis
  - Recurrent EN (erythema multiforme)

"Thought is the wind, knowledge the sail, and mankind the vessel."

Augustus Hare

FEVER OF UNKNOWN ORIGIN (FUO)

➢ Definition: "………. an illness that lasts at least 3 weeks in a patient with temperature greater than 38°C (101.0 °F) on several occasions and whose diagnosis remains uncertain despite having been evaluated in a hospital for at least 1 week".

MKSAP 16, Infectious disease 2012, page 52.

➢ Several different definitions

Type of FUO	Temperature °C (°F)	Duration	Diagnosis remains uncertain
o Classic	> 38.3 (101.0)	> 3 wk	> 1 wk hospital investigation
o Modified classic	> 38.0 (100.4)	> 3 wk	> 3 days hospital investigation, or > 2 outpatient visits with tests not showing cause
o Health-care associated	> 38.0 (100.4)	> 3 days	Hospitalized patient Acute care Infection not present (or incubating on admission)
o Immune-deficient	> 38.0 (100.4))	-	> 3 days appropriate (includes 2 days for incubation of cultures)
o HIV (confirmed)-related	> 38.0 (100.4))	> 3 wk in outpatients, or > 3 days in patients	

SO YOU WANT TO BE AN INFECTIOUS DISEASE EXPERT!

- Give 3 types of **hereditary periodic fever syndrome** in which there is > 14 days without fever between recurrent episodes of FUO.

    - HIDS (hyperimmunoglobulin D syndrome)
        - Autosomal recessive
        - Clinical
            - Lymphadenopathy
            - Abdomen
                - Pain
                - Diarrhea
            - Joints
                - Pain
            - Skin
                - Maculopapulary rash
            - Serum
                - ↑ IgA, ↑ IgD

    - TRAPS (tumor-necrosis factor receptor-1 associated periodic syndrome)
        - Autosomal dominant
        - Clinical
            - Eyes
                - Periorbital edema
                - Conjunctivitis
            - Abdomen
                - Pain
            - Joints
                - Arthritis
            - Skin
                - Red patches
            - Testes
                - Pain

    - Muckle-Wells syndrome
        - Autosomal dominant
        - Clinical
            - Ears ↓ sensoneural hearing
            - Abdomen pain
            - Joints arthralgia arthritis
            - Skin urticarial
            - Amyloidosis

    - FMF (familial Mediterranean fever)
        - Autosomal recessive
        - Clinical
            - Chest
                - Pain
            - Abdomen
                - Pain
            - Joints
                - Arthritis
            - Serositis
            - Skin
                - Foot rash

- Perform a focused physical examination for fever of unknown origin.

Temporal artery
- Temporal arteritis

Sinus disease
- Chronic sinusitis
- Wegeners granulomatosis

Teeth/ Jaw
- Abscess
- Osteomyelitis

Painful neck lumps
- Thyroiditis (+ thyrotoxic)
- Infections in lymph nodes

Lymphadenopathy
- Infections, especially viral
- Malignancy
- Granulomatous disease (e.g. sarcoidosis)

Tender/weak shoulder/hip muscles
- Polymyalgia
- Polymyositis

Hepatomegaly
- Hepatitis (esp. alcoholic, granulomatosis)
- Malignancy (esp. secondary)

Heart
- Pericarditis
- Infective endocarditis (esp. tricuspid)
- Repeated PE
- Dressier's syndrome
- Atrial myxoma

Aorta
- Mycotic aneurysm
- Inflammatory

Splinter hemorrhages
- Infective endocarditis
- Vasculitis
- Sepsis

Splenomegaly
- Sepsis
- Chronic liver disease
- Blood malignancy
- Sarcoidosis

Renal mass
- Cancer
- Abscess

Pain
- Bone, muscle (infection, malignancy, inflammation)

Perianal lesions
- Sepsis
- Crohn's

Joints
- Infection
- Connective tissue disease
- Rheumatological disease

Skin sepsis

Leg swelling/ tenderness
- Deep vein thrombosis
- Cellulitis

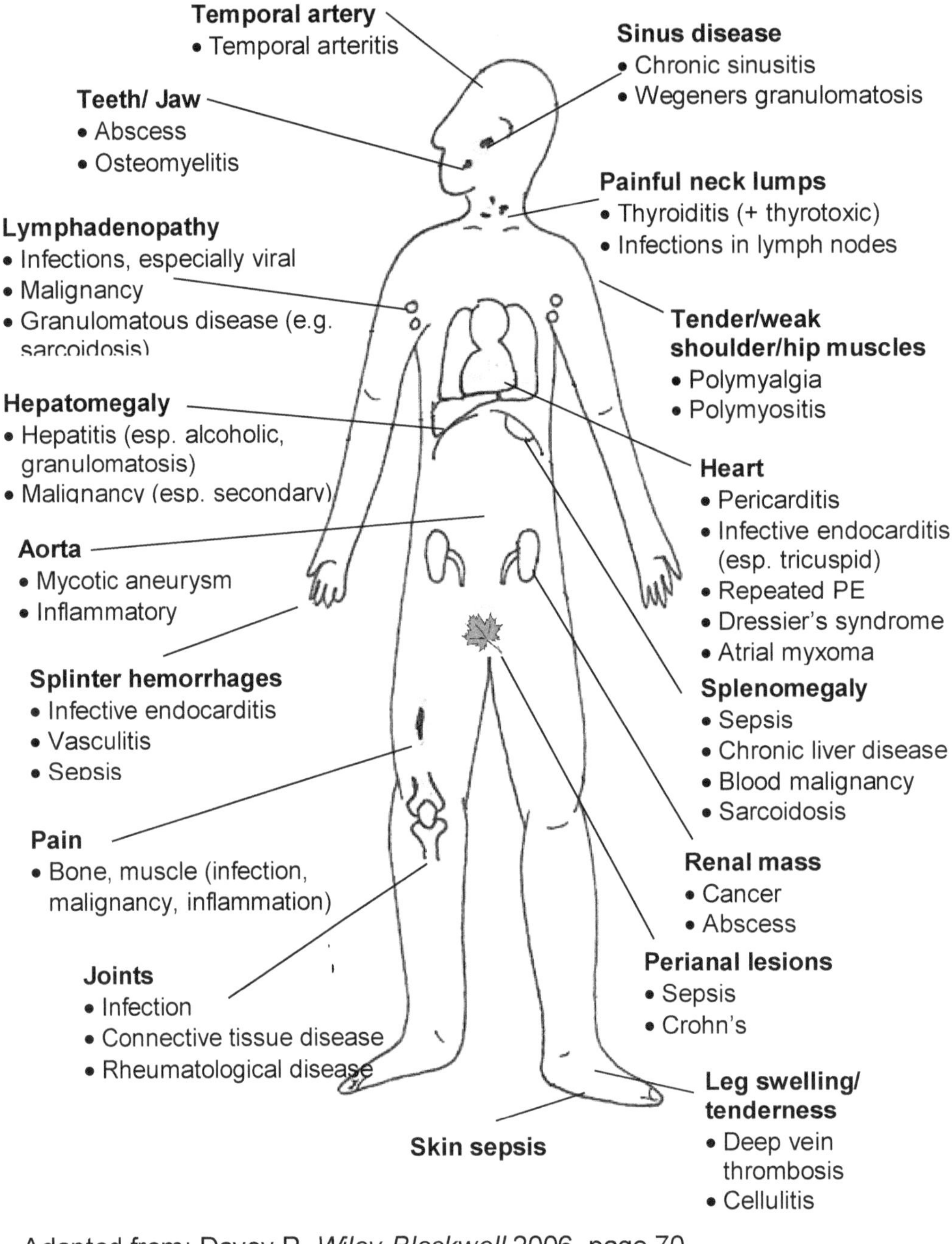

Adapted from: Davey P. *Wiley-Blackwell* 2006, page 70.

- Give the common causes of fever of unknown origin.

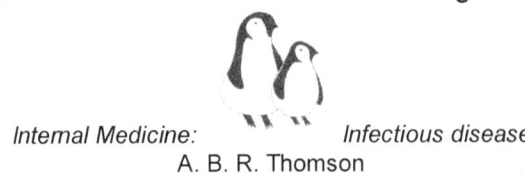

Internal Medicine: *Infectious disease*
A. B. R. Thomson

- ➤ Infections
  - o Most common cause; common illness presenting in an atypical manner
  - o Most common infectious causes
    - – Lung
      - ▪ Tuberculosis
    - – Heart
      - ▪ Infective endocarditis
    - – GI / GU
      - ▪ Abdominal / pelvic abscess
  - o Infection (extensive search in HIV infections) EBV, CMV, HBV / HCV
- ➤ Neoplasms (infiltration)
  - o Lymphoma
  - o Solid tumors (gastrointestinal tract, liver, renal cell, sarcoma)
  - o Leukemia, and other hematological tumors
  - o Atrial myxoma
  - o Inflammatory - IBD, connective-tissue diseases
  - o Vascular – pulmonary emboli
  - o Iatrogenic – drug-induced (malignant hypertrophy)
  - o Congenital – familial Mediterranean fever
- ➤ Connective tissue disease (autoimmune)
  - o Temporal arteritis/polymyalgia rheumatica
  - o Polyarteritis nodosa
  - o Systemic lupus erythematosus (SLE)
  - o Still disease
  - o Iatrogenic (drugs, toxin)
  - o Special considerations
    - – Heart
      - ▪ Endocarditis
      - ▪ HACEK
        - – Haemophilus aphrophilis
        - – Actinobacillus actinomycetem comitans
        - – Cardiobacterium hominis
        - – Eikenella corrodes
        - – Kingella kingae
    - – Blood

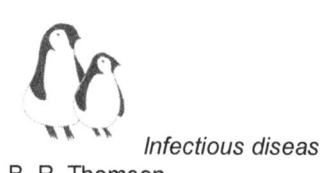

Internal Medicine: *Infectious disease*
A. B. R. Thomson

- Lymphoproliferative disorders
- Hematoma
  - Lung
    - PE (pulmonary embolus)
    - TB
  - Endocrine
    - Hypo- hyperthyroidism
    - Pheochromocytoma
- ○ Factitious
- ○ Habitual hyperthermia
- ○ Hereditary periodic fever syndromes

Ideopathic (50%)

Adapted from: Jugovic PJ, et al. *Saunders/ Elsevier* 2004, pages 37 to 39.

➢ Bacteremia in febrile patients

Risk Factors	PLR	NLR
○ Renal failure	4.6	0.8
○ Hospitalization for trauma	3.0	NS
○ Intravenous drug use	2.9	NS
○ Previous stroke	2.8	NS
○ Poor functional performance	3.6	0.6
○ Rapid fatal disease (<1 mo)	2.7	NS

Abbreviation: NLR, negative likelihood ratio; PLR positive likelihood ratio

Note that some clinical features are not included, because their PLR was < 2. These include: age 50 years or more and diabetes mellitus.

Adapted from: McGee SR. *Saunders/Elsevier* 2007, Box 16-2, page 180.

- Give 5 conditions which in the patient with fever of unknown origin, **a bone marrow aspiration** may be useful to diagnose.

  - ○ Malignancy
    - Leukemia
    - Lymphoma
    - Bone cancer

  - ○ Infection

Internal Medicine: *Infectious disease*
A. B. R. Thomson

- TB
- Malaria
- Kala- azar
- Brucellosis

- Take a directed history and perform a focused physical examination for **postoperative (post-op) fever**.

    o Post-operative risk factors /complications
        - Age > 50 years
        - Pre-existing cognitive dysfunction
        - Depression perioperative derangements
        - > 5 prescribed medications postoperatively
        - Use of anti-cholinergics preoperatively
        - Cardiopulmonary bypass
        - ICU setting

    o Wound
        - Inflammation
        - Leakage

    o IV site
        - Cellulitis

    o Limbs
        - Thrombophlebitis

    o Medications / Blood products
        - Medications (previous / new)
        - Blood product reactions
        - Allergies

    o Lung
        - Atelectasis
        - Aspiration
        - Pneumonia
        - Pulmonary embolus
    o GI
        - Ileus
        - Perforation
        - Abscess

    o UTI

Adapted from: Jugovic PJ, et al. *Saunders/ Elsevier* 2004, pages 76 to 78.

The presence of a **skin rash** in the patient **with fever** helps to narrow the likely

Internal Medicine: *Infectious disease*
A. B. R. Thomson

conditions causing a fever.

- Give causes of fever and rash.
- Specific
    - Vesicobullous
        - Herpes viruses (particularly varicella zoster virus)
        - Coxsackie
        - Enterovirus
        - Mycoplasma

    - Petechia, purpura or skin hemorrhage
        - Meningococcal septicemia
        - Staphylococcus aureus
        - Viral hemorrhagic fevers
        - Typhus
        - Leptospirosis
        - Gram-negative septicemia

    - Nodular rash
        - Erythema nodosum

    - Diffuse generalized erythema
        - Scalded skin syndrome
        - Toxic shock syndrome
            - Usually due to staphylococcal colonization of tampons
            - Symptoms during or shortly after menstruation
            - Fever, hypotension, shock
            - Scarlet skin eruption
            - Desquamation
            - Multi organ failure

    - Maculo-papular rashes (non-specific)
        - Drug reaction
        - Infection
        - Self-limiting viral infections
        - HIV seroconversion
        - Dengue fever

Adapted from: Davey P. *Wiley-Blackwell* 2006, page 72.
Performance Characteristics for Patients with Fever

Physical examination	PLR	NLR
o Urinary catheter	2.4	NS
o Central venous line	2.0	NS

Abbreviation: NLR, negative likelihood ratio; PLR positive likelihood ratio

Note that numerous findings are not listed here, because their PLR is < 2. These include: Temperature $\geq$ 38.5 °C, tachycardia, respiratory rate > 20/min, hypotension, acute abdomen and confusion or depressed sensorium.

Adapted from: McGee SR. *Saunders/Elsevier* 2007, Box 16-2, page 180.

Performance characteristics of prognosis of clinical findings in fever > 39°C.

Finding	PLR	NLR
➢ Temperature > 39 °C		
o Predicting hospital mortality in patients with pontine hemorrhage	23.7	0.4
➢ Hypothermia		
o Predicting hospital mortality		
- From pump failure in patients with heart failure	6.7	NS
- In patients with pneumonia	3.5	NS
- In patients with bacteremia	3.3	NS

Abbreviation: NLR, negative likelihood ratio; NS, not significant; PLR positive likelihood ratio

Adapted from: McGee SR. *Saunders/Elsevier* 2007, Box 16-3, page 182.

"Let's see if there is mechanistic information that we can tease out."

Grandad

SEPTIC SHOCK

Internal Medicine: *Infectious disease*
A. B. R. Thomson

➢ Definition: "…. an exaggerated inflammatory response to an infections stimulus ….. characterized by a severe catabolic reaction, widespread endothelial dysfunction, and release of inflammation agents" (MKSAP 16 2013, Pulmonary, page 82)
   o MR (mortality rate)
      - SIR (systemic inflammatory response syndrome) includes
         ▪ ↑ T (temperature)
         ▪ ↑ HR (heart rate)
         ▪ ↑ RR (respiratory rate)
         ▪ ↓ WBC (neutropenia)
      - Sepsis is SIR plus suspected infection
      - 20% for each sepsis-induced dysfunction
      - 17% if appropriate antibiotic are used

• Give the definition of FUO (fever of unknown origin), sepsis and SIRS (systemic inflammatory response syndrome).

Response to infection	Endpoints to define sepsis or SIRS
o ↑, ↓ T	– > 38.0 °C (100.4 F), or – < 36.0 °C (96.8 F)
o ↑ HR	– > 90 bpm
o ↑ RR	– > 20 / min, or – a PCO_2 < 32 mmHg
o ↑ WBC	– > 12,000 / µL, or – < 4000 / µL plus 10% bands
o Sepsis	– Known or suspected infection (positive cultures not necessary), plus – ≥ 2 criteria above

o SIRS (systemic inflammatory response syndrome)	– ≥ 2 criteria above
	– Severe sepsis
	  ▪ Sepsis-induced hypotension / hypoperfusion
	– Septic shock
	  ▪ Sepsis-induced hyotension / hypoperfusion despite appropriate resuscitation with fluids

➢ Pathophysiology

- Give the changes in CO (cardiac output), PCWP (pulmonary capillary wedge pressure) and SVR (systemic vascular resistance) in 4 shock syndromes.

Shock syndrome	CO	PCWP	SVR	Associations
o Cardiogenic	↓	↑	↑	Signs of HF (heart failure)
o Hypovolemic	↓	↓	↑	Signs of blood loss / volume loss
o Obstructive	↓	↓	↑	PE (pulmonary embolism) Tension pneumothorax Cardiac tamponade
o Anaphylactic	↑	N	↓	Skin – Rash – Urticaria – Angioedma Lung – Wheeze – Stridor
o Septic*	↑ / ↓		↓	↑ T, ↑ HR, ↑ RR, ↓ aPCo$_2$, ↑ / ↓ WBC

*Early ↑ and then ↓ CO

Abbreviations: HR, heart rate; T, temperature; WBC, white blood cells

➤ Laboratory

- In the setting of sepsis, give 3 clinical / lab' changes suggestive of hypotension / hypoperfusion.

  o Lactic acidosis

  o Acute ↓ LOC (loss of consciousness or change in mental function)

  o Acute kidney injury (AKI)

➤ Classification of Sepsis, Severe Sepsis and Septic Shock

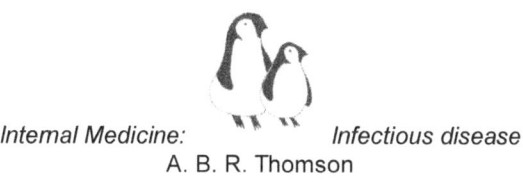

Internal Medicine: *Infectious disease*
A. B. R. Thomson

Clinical Staging	Diagnostic Criteria
o Sepsis	– Clinical evidence suggestive of infection plus:
	– Signs of a systemic inflammatory response to infection (≥2 of the following):
	– Tachypnea (>20 breaths/min or $PaCO_2$ <32 mm Hg [<4.3 kPa])
	– Tachycardia (>90 beats//min)
	– Hyperthemia (>38° C)
	– WBC > 12 x 10^9 Cells/L, or <4 x 10^9 Cells/L, or >10% immature (band) forms
o Severe sepsis	– Sepsis with hypotension (systolic blood pressure <90 mmHg or a 40 mm Hg decrease from baseline in the absence of other causes)
	– Organ dysfunction and perfusion abnormalities such as:
	▪ Oliguria: <0.5 mL/kg for at least 1 h in patients with urinary catheters
	▪ ↑Plasma lactate (>normal upper limit)
	▪ Altered mental status
o Septic shock	– Severe sepsis as defined above, despite adequate fluid resuscitation
	Note: patients who are on pressor agents may not be hypotensive

Reproduced with permission: Therapeutics Choices. Sixth Edition. Ottawa, *Canada: Canadian Pharmacist Association* 2012, Table 1, page 1490.

➤ Clinical
  o Pulse rate (PR) and fever (PR normally increases 8 bpm for each 1°C increase in body temperature)
    - Lower pulse than expected for temperature
      ▪ Typhoid fever
      ▪ Brucellosis
      ▪ Meningitis
    - Higher pulse than expected for temp'
      ▪ Polyarteritis (in fact, fever may be only slight)
  o Fever plus purpura
    - Septicemia
    - Hematological disorder

Internal Medicine: *Infectious disease*
A. B. R. Thomson

- Hemorrhagic exanthemas
- Remittent
  - Temperature raised throughout the day
  - Difference between maximum and minimum temp' is $>2^0$F
- Intermittent
  - High peaks with return to normal at some point each day
  - Suggests abscess, septicemia, malaria
- Continuous
  - Temperature raised throughout the day
  - Difference between maximum and minimum temp' is $< 2^0$F
  - Suggests
    - SBE
    - Viral pneumonia
    - Military TB
    - Typhoid fever
- Relapsing (aka undulating)
  - Periods of normal temperature between periods of high temp'
  - Suggestive of
    - Brucellosis
    - Spirochaetal infection
    - Reticulosis
    - Bite and scratch fevers

➢ Organs

- o CNS   – Delirium

- o Lung   – ARDS (acute respiratory stress syndrome)
  - Pneumothorax (from mechanical ventilation)
  - Aspiration pneumonitis / pneumonia
  - Pleural effusions
  - Nosocomial pneumonia
  - PE (pulmonary embolism)

- o Heart   – Pericardial effusions

- o Kidney   – Acute renal failure
  - pH, fluid and electrolyte disturbances

- o Blood   – DIC (disseminated intravascular coagulation)
  - Thrombocytopenia
  - DVT (deep vein thrombosis), +/- PE

Internal Medicine: *Infectious disease*
A. B. R. Thomson

- o GI tract
  - – Malnutrition
  - – Stress ulceration
  - – Gastroparesis
  - – Hepatic dysfunction
  - – ↑ risk of drug AEs (adverse effects, from ↓ hepatic metabolism of certain drugs)

The septic patient

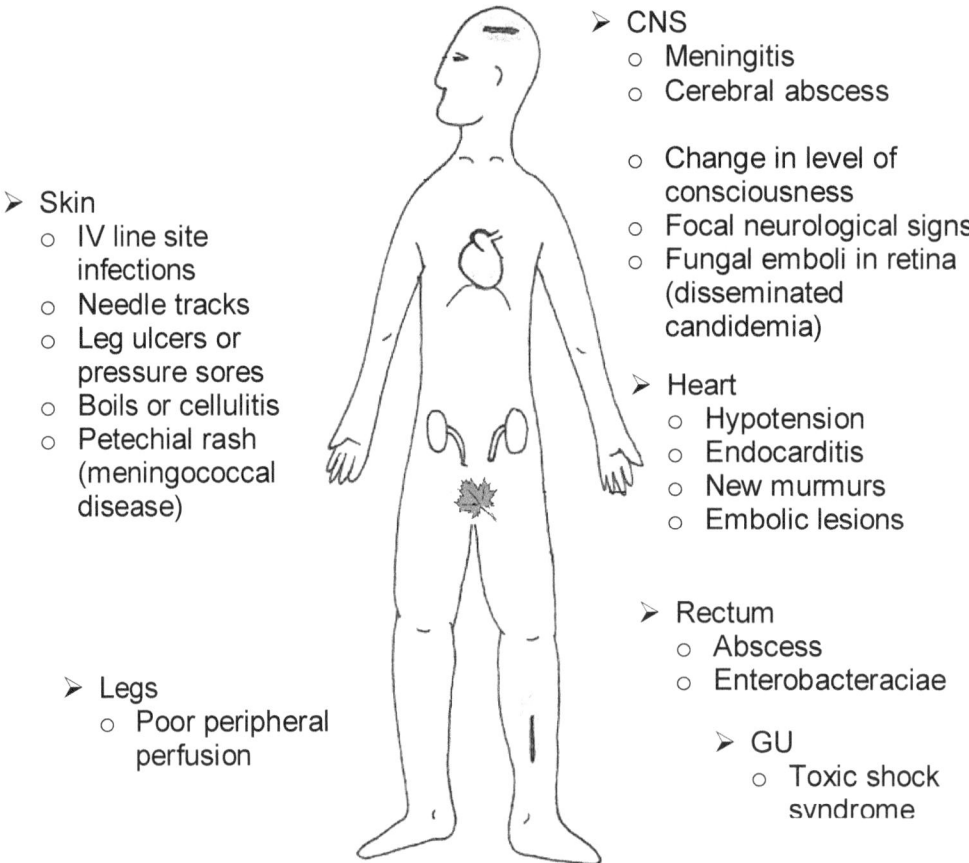

> CNS
> o Meningitis
> o Cerebral abscess
>
> o Change in level of consciousness
> o Focal neurological signs
> o Fungal emboli in retina (disseminated candidemia)

> Skin
> o IV line site infections
> o Needle tracks
> o Leg ulcers or pressure sores
> o Boils or cellulitis
> o Petechial rash (meningococcal disease)

> Heart
> o Hypotension
> o Endocarditis
> o New murmurs
> o Embolic lesions

> Rectum
> o Abscess
> o Enterobacteraciae

> GU
> o Toxic shock syndrome

> Legs
> o Poor peripheral perfusion

Adapted from: Davey P. *Wiley-Blackwell* 2006, page 296.

Useful background: Reasons why a senior may have urinary incontinence ("**DRIP**"

- o **D**elirium/diabetes mellitus
- o **R**estricted mobility/retention

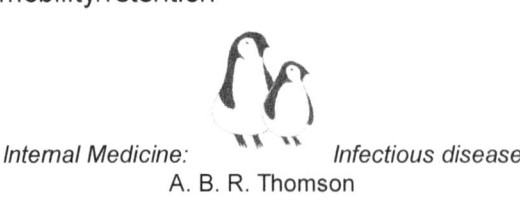

Internal Medicine: *Infectious disease*
A. B. R. Thomson

- o Infections (UTI)/Impaction of stool
- o **P**sychological / pills (long acting sedatives, diuretics, anticholinergic agents)

Source: Jugovic PJ, et al. *Saunders/ Elsevier* 2004, page 30.

o Ceftaroline	–	Community-acquired non-MRSA pneumonia
o Daptomycin	–	S. aureus bacteremia when there is resistance to
	–	Severe skin infections; vancomycin, i.e. MIC (minimal inhibitory concentration > 2 mcg/mL
o Doripenem	–	Complicated
	▪	UTI / pyelonephritis
	▪	Intraabdominal infections
o Linezolid	–	VRE (Vancomycin-resistant enterococcus faecium) infections
	–	Nosocomial skin infections
	–	Community-acquired pneumonia (CAP)
o Telavancin	–	Complicated skin infections
o Tigecycline	–	Complicated
	▪	Skin infection
	▪	Intraabdominal infection
	–	CAP

- o Insulin to correct hyperglycemia, to maintain blood glucose < 10 mmol/L
- o Sedation-intermittent or bolus (not continuous)
- o Compression devises
- o Anti-coagulation with heparin
- o IV PPI prophylaxis vs. stress ulcers
- o Dialysis, as needed
- o Treat cause / complications, e.g. lactic acidosis

Internal Medicine: *Infectious disease*
A. B. R. Thomson

Clinical Gems

- o About 1/3 of persons treated for smoke inhalation from fires have associated **cyanide toxicity**.
- o **Angioedema** may occur
  - As a part of anaphylaxis resulting from activation of IgE on the surface of mast cells and basophils
  - Not as a part of anaphylaxis (not mediated by IgE release), such as from
    - Brucellosis
    - Trauma
    - Infection
    - Drugs (e.g. ACE inhibitors)
    - C1 esterase (inhibitor) deficiency
    - Possibly associated with lymphoproliferative disorder

- Give the treatment for a **septic shock**.

  - o Treat the underlying cause(s)

  - o Heart
    - CVP (central venous pressure), 8-12 mm Hg
      - IV fluids to correct CVP
      - May require 10-20 L/day
    - MAP (mean arterial pressure) > 65 mm Hg
      - Vasoactive agents (Norepinephrine or dopamine (vasopressin) to correct MAP (if correction of CVP not sufficient)

  - o Lung
    - Supplemental O_2
    - Mechanical ventilation
    - Packed RBC for S cvo_2 < 70%, to maintain hematocrit > 30%
    - Inotropic agents if S cvo_2 < 70% despite RBC transfusion
    - Sv CO_2
      - Hct (hematocrit)
        - < 30% - transfusion ⎤ to correct
        - ≥ 30% - dopamine or ⎥ $SvCO_2$ once
        dobutamine (inotropes) ⎦ CAP and MAP corrected
    - ARDS (acute respiratory distress syndrome)
      - Mechanical ventilation 6 mL/kg and plateau pressures
  - o Antibiotics
    - Early use of appropriate antibiotics, using

Internal Medicine: *Infectious disease*
A. B. R. Thomson

combination therapy

- o Endocrine
  - Blood sugar
  - Corticosteroids
    - Low dose if systolic pressure < 90 mm Hg despite IV fluids or vasopressors
    - Do not use high-dose, or for toxic shock syndrome

- o Renal
  - Maintain UO (urine output) > 0.5 mL/kg per hr
  - Us above measures of fluids, vasopressors, steroids

- o Empiric antibiotics (for sepsis; please see definition above)

- Community-acquired infection	▪ Cephalosporin or carbapenem ± vancomycin

- Healthcare-associated infection	▪ Especially patients who had received
	  - Antibiotics
	  - Immunosuppressants
	  - Chemotherapy
	▪ Vancomycin plus
	▪ β-lactam (anti-pseudomonas), plus
	▪ Fluoroquinolone or aminoglycoside

MAP = (SBP + 1DBP)/ 3

Abbreviations: DBP, diastolic blood pressure; MAP, mean arterial pressure; SBP, systolic blood pressure

---

Pearl and Gem

- o For septic shock, use low-dose, not high-dose corticosteroids
- o For toxic shock syndrome, do <u>not</u> use corticosteroids

---

Toxic Shock Syndrome

➢ Definition

- o Shock syndrome, exfoliating rash, "packing" infected by Staphylococcus aureus and group A β-hemolytic streptococci

Internal Medicine:　　　　*Infectious disease*
A. B. R. Thomson

- o "packing"
    - Tampoon for menstrual bleeding
    - Nasal packing
    - Wound packing
    - Abscess

- o The body temperature is often > 38.9°C (102.0 F, and systolic blood pressure < 90 mm Hg

- ➢ Treatment
    - o Toxic shock syndrome
        - Empiric
            - Carbapenem or penicllin, plus
            - β-lactamase inhibitor, plus
            - Clinidamycin
        - IV immune globulin
        - Once organism found clindamycin plus nafcillin

    Note: do **not** use corticosteroids

FLUSHING

- Perform a directed physical examination for flushing.

    - o Anxiety
    - o Skin disease
        - Acne
        - Rosacea
        - Photosensitive dermatitis

    - o Drugs
        - Alcohol
        - Ca^{2+} channel blockers

    - o Food
        - Scombroid poisoning

    - o Tumor
        - Carcinoid tumors
            - Medullary thyroid cancer
            - Systemic mastocytosis

Note that skin conditions or self-limiting infections may cause sweating without flushing

Adapted from: Davey P. *Wiley-Blackwell* 2006, page 54.

Internal Medicine: *Infectious disease*
A. B. R. Thomson

CLASS A BIOTERRORISM AGENTS

- o Anthrax
- o Smallpox
- o Plague
- o Botulism
- o Tularemia
- o Viral hemorrhagic fever

Anthrax

➢ Definition
- o "Anthrax infection is caused by the bacterium Bacillus anthracis.....to describe the destructive block eochar associated with cutaneous disease. This gram-positive, 'box cow' – shaped, aerobic, non-motile bacillus is found in soil worldwide, predominantly in agricultural areas". (MKSAP 16, Infectious disease 2012, page 57)
- o Spore as inhaled, ingested, or contact the skin

➢ Clinical
- o Pulmonary anthrax
  - May become fulminant and cause death
  - Diagnosis
    - Culture ⎱ sputum, blood tissue
    - PCR ⎰
    - Chest X-ray, wide mediastinum (hemorrhagic lymphadenopathy)
  - Treatment
    - For 60 days, IV for 2 wk, then po for 7 wk
    - Ciprofloxacin, or
    - Doxycycline plus1 or 2 of
      - Penicillin
      - Ampicillin
- o Cutaneous anthax
  - Must be treated, since treated, since otherwise mortality rate is ~ 15% due to secondary bacteremic spread
- o GI anthax
  - Must also be treated because of mortality rate of ~ 40%

Please see standard textbook or recent reviews such as UptoDate or MKSAP 16, Infectious disease 2012, Table 30, page 56.

Internal Medicine:　　　　*Infectious disease*
A. B. R. Thomson

➢ Prophylaxis

   o Antibiotics
     – Ciprofloxacin, or
     – Doxycycline

   o Antrax vaccine

Small pox (aka Variola)

➢ Clinical   o A human only infecting mucosa of mouth / pharynx
     – Face
     – Arms
     – Hands
     – Legs
     – Feet

   o Synchronous (for any part of the body, e.g. face, skin lesion are all at the same stage of maturity)

   o Macules → papules → vesicles → pustules → scabs / crusts

   o Contagious until scabs / crusts have cleared

   o When variola affects the eyes → keratitis → ulcers of cornea → blindness

   o Mortality rate ~ 30% (variola minor, MR < 1%)

• Give the clinical features which help to distinguish the rash of chicken pox (varicella) from smallpox (variola).

Disease	Initial site	Spreads (distribution)	Stage of maturation at one site
o Chickenpox	Trunk	Periphery (centripedal)	Asynchronous
o Smallpox	Buccal mucosa pharynx	Face, arms / legs, hand / feet (centraifacal)	Synchronous

➢ Diagnosis   o PCR assays

   o Contact CDC (Centres for Disease Control and Prevention)
   http://emergency.cdc.gov/agent/smallpox/diagnosis/#diagnosis

➢ Treatment   o Cidofovir

   o Vaccination
     – Active post-exposure administration to patient
     – Close contacts ("ring vaccination")

Plague

- ➢ Causes / associations
  - ○ Yersinia pestis
  - ○ Gram-negative coccobacillus (bipolar staining, shape of a safety pin)
  - ○ Infects rats / cats → flea bite in humans

- ➢ Clinical
  - ○ Purulent lymphadenitis near site of flea bite
  - ○ Pneumonic
    - – Primary
    - – Secondary, from
      - ▪ Prurulent nodes
      - ▪ Septicemia
  - ○ Septicemia
  - ○ Mortality rate without treatment ~ 100%

- ➢ Diagnosis
  - ○ Gram stain
    - – Blood
    - – Sputum

- ➢ Treatment
  - ○ Symptomatic
    - – Antibiotics
      - ▪ Streptomycin or gentamycin, or
      - ▪ Fluoroquinolone, or
      - ▪ Doxycycline for 10 days
    - – Isolation respiratory droplet precautions for 2 days after start of antibiotics
  - ○ Asymptomatic contacts
    - – Prophylactic fluoroquinolone or doxycycline for 7 days
  - ○ Vaccination
    - – Not available

Botulism

- ➢ Causes / associations
  - ○ Clostridium botulinium, anaerobic gram-positive spore-forming bacillus
  - ○ Release of highly lethal toxin (blocks Ach [acetylcholine] mediated neurotransmission)
  - ○ Inhalation, ingestion, skin contact

- ➤ Clinical
  - o "4 D's"
  - o Descending flaccid paralyses (diaphragm involvement → respiratory failure)
  - o No-fever
    - – Mental changes
- ➤ Diagnosis
  - o Identify toxin (skin, stool, vomitus, contaminating food)
- ➤ Treatment
  - o Rapid use of antitoxin (trivalent, derived from horses)
  - o Limitation-does not reverse toxin-inhibited neurotransmission of Ach

Tularemia

- ➤ Causes / associations
  - o Gram-negative coccobacilllus, Francisella tularensis the organism affects arthropod (ticks) which bites human
  - o Also transmitted by inhalation or ingestion

- ➤ Clinical
  - o Pneumonia → respiration or ingestion
  - o Typhoid-like illness
  - o Septicemia → septic shock
  - o Mortality rate ~ 30%

- ➤ Diagnosis
  - o Serology
  - o Culture (too slow)
  - o Tissue
    - – Immunofluorescence
    - – PCR
    - – Granulomatous infiltration
    - – Infiltration
      - ▪ Lobar
      - ▪ Subsegmental
      - ▪ Oval
    - – Pleural effusions
    - – Hilar lymphadenopathy
  - o Chest x-ray

- ➤ Treatment
  - o Streptomycin, or
  - o Gentamycin for 7 to 14 days
  - o Post-exposure prophylaxis
    - – Ciprofloxacin, or
    - – Doxycycline
  - o Vaccination: not available

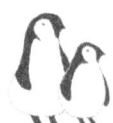

TRAVEL MEDICINE

- Give the causes of **fever in the returned traveler**.

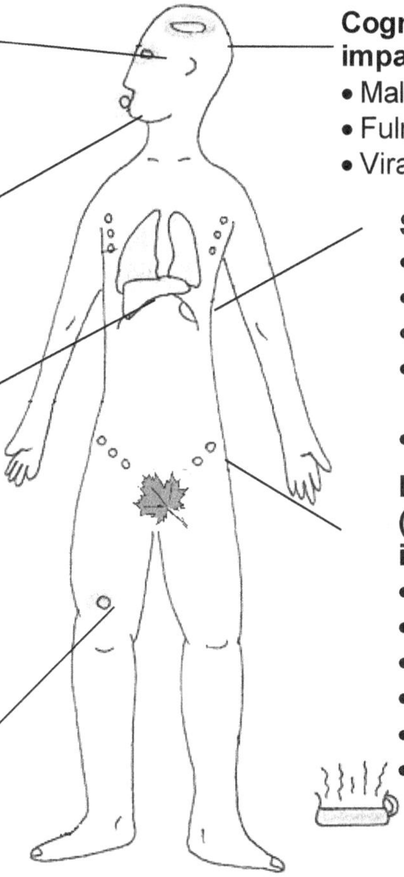

Jaundice
- Hepatitis
- Malaria
- Leptospirosis
- Yellow fever

Cognitive impairment/delirium
- Malaria
- Fulminant hepatic failure
- Viral encephalitis

Vomiting
- GI pathogens
- Malaria

Spenomegaly
- Malaria
- Typhoid
- Brucellosis
- Visceral leishmaniasis
- Rickettsial diseases

Hepatomegaly
- Amebic liver abscess (often tender)
- Hepatitis
- Typhoid
- Malaria
- Leptospirosis

Lymphadenopathy (common in many infections)
- Rickettsial infections
- HIV
- Plague (localized, tender)
- Brucellosis
- Filariasis
- Visceral leishmaniasis

Diarrhea
- GI pathogens

Skin lesion

Rose spots	- Typhoid
Eschar	- Tick and scrub typhus - Anthrax
Petechiae/hemorrhage	- Viral hemorrhagic fevers - Leptospirosis
Maculopapular	- Dengue, tick typhus, syphilis, arboviral infections, leptospirosis, HIV
Chancre	- African trypanosomiasis

Adapted from: Davey P. *Wiley-Blackwell*, 2006 page 76.

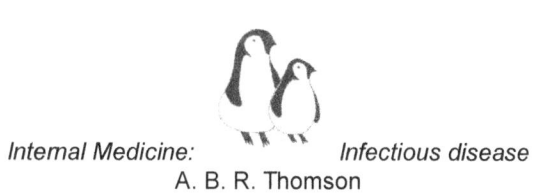

- ➢ Causes / associations
  - ○ Bacteria
    - – Typhoid fever
      - ▪ Salmonella enerica serotype Typhi (aka S. typhi)
    - – Traveller's diarrhea
      - ▪ Multiple organisms
    - – Brucellosis
      - ▪ Brucella
  - ○ Viruses
    - – Dengue fever
      - ▪ Flaviviridae (DENV-1 to DENV-4)
    - – Mononucleosis syndrome
      - ▪ CMV (cytomegalovirus)
      - ▪ EBV (Epstein-Barr virus)
    - – Hepatitis A virus
  - ○ Parasites
    - – Malaria
      - ▪ Plasmodium species
  - ○ Rickettsia
    - – Rickettsia typhi
    - – R. prowazekii
  - ○ Fungi
    - – Histoplasma capsulatum
    - – Coccidioides spaces
    - – Penicilum marneffei

Brucellosis

- ➢ Cause
  - ○ Gram-negative coccobacillus Brucella species
  - ○ Inhalation
  - ○ Ingestion
    - – Unpasturized milk
    - – Undercooked meat
  - ○ Skin direct contact

- ➢ Clinical
  - ○ Night sweats
  - ○ CNS neuropsychiatric symptoms
  - ○ Heart endocarditis

➢ Diagnosis

     o Culture
       – Blood
       – Bone marrow

     o Serological tests

➢ Treatment

     o Doxycycline plus rifampin plus streptomycin or gentamycin

Dengue Fever

➢ Causes / associations

     o Viruses of the Flaviviridae (DENV-1 to -4) family are carried by mosquitos

➢ Clinical

     o Febrile illness
       – A second "saddleback" febile pattern may develop)

     o Headache retro-orbital pain

     o Bleeding
       – Purpura
       – Conjunctival injection

     o Back pain
       – "breakbone fever" affecting lumbosarcral region

     o Rash (measles-like) as the fever subsides → petecliae on backs of hands and feet (exterior surfaces)

     o Liver failure

➢ Diagnosis

     o Real-time reverse transcriptase PCR (polymerase chain reaction) of blood

     o Serologic testing of serum, acute and convalsecent

     o ELISA test

➢ Treatment and vaccination

     o None

     o Supportive cure only

Internal Medicine: *Infectious disease*
A. B. R. Thomson

Malaria

➤ Causes / associations
- o Plasmodium species parasites, transmitted by bite of female Anopheles mosquito
- o Parasite enters RBCs
- o Multiple thrombosis occur in small blood vessels
- o P. falciparum
  - – Common species
  - – Severe risk of choroquine resistance
  - – Potentially lethal

➤ Clinical
- o CNS
  - – Δ LOC (level of consciousness)
  - – Seizures
- o Liver
  - – Hepatic failure
- o Kidney
  - – AKI
  - – Metabolic acidosis
- o Endocrine
  - – Hypoglycemia
- o Blood
  - – DIC (disseminated intravascular)
  - – Thrombocytopenia coagulation
  - – Hemolysis (intravascular)

➤ Diagnosis
- o Peripheral blood smear
- o PCR, and other molecular technique to determine species

➤ Treatment
- o Chemoprophylaxis for endemic areas
  - – Plasmodium falciparum
    - ▪ Chloroquine-sensitive
    - ▪ Chloroquine-resistant

	Drug	Dose	P. vivax	
			Treatment stat & travel	
			Start before	Stop after
o	Mefloquine	250 mg qw	1-2 wk	4 wk
o	Atovaquone / proguanil	250 mg / 100 mg OD	1-2 d	7 d
o	Doxycycline	100 mg OD	1-2 d	4 wk

Note

Internal Medicine: *Infectious disease*
A. B. R. Thomson

- o Choice of chemo-prophylaxis depends upon destination
- o Unless absolute essential, pregnant women should not place themselves and then unborn child at risk and travel to an area here malaria is present
- o Please see standard textbooks for further recommendations about chemoprophylaxis fo malaria. Also see http://www.nc.cdc.gov/travel/yellowbook/2012/chapter-3-infectious-disease-related-to-travel/malaria.htm

It is recommended that a pregnant women **not** travel to an area in which malaria is endemic, so as to prevent the morbidity of this infection to the mother and child. However, in the event that travel is essential, give the recommended prophylaxis.

- o Chloroquine sensitive   – Chloroquine 500 mg OW
- o Chloroquine resistant   – Mefloquine 250 mg OW

Abbreviation: OW, once weekly

Rickettsioses

- ➢ Causes / associations
  - o Intracellular gram-negative bacteria transmitted by fleas, lice, mites, ticks; e.g.
    - – Rickettsia typhi fleas vector
    - – R. prowazekii body lice

- ➢ Clinical
  - o Febrile illness
  - o Rash
    - – Maculopapular
    - – Vesicular
    - – Petechial

- ➢ Diagnosis
  - o Culture of involved skin
  - o Biopsy immunohistochemistry
  - o PCR

- ➢ Treatment
  - o Doxycycline
  - o No vaccine available

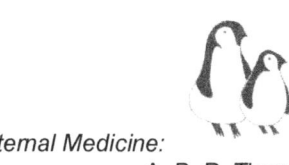

Internal Medicine: *Infectious disease*
A. B. R. Thomson

Typhoid Fever

- ➢ Causes / associations
  - o Salmonella enterica serotype typhi (aka Salmonella typhi)
  - o Consumption of food and water contaminated by human feces

- ➢ Clinical
  - o Fever "enteric" everyday for 4-8 wk
  - o Diarrhea
  - o Bleeding / bowel perforation (2 to 3 wk after beginning of infection)
  - o Rose spot rash (1 to 4 wk after beginning of infection)
  - o High risk of chronic state in person with cholelithiasis

- ➢ Diagnosis
  - o Culture
    - Stoll
    - Urine
    - Blood
    - Bone marrow
  - o Serology molecular methods have replaced traditional Wodal test for anti-O and –H antigens

- ➢ Treatment
  - o Empiric therapy of choice is changing because of fluoroquine resistance
  - o Fluoroquine or ceftriaxone
  - o Typhoic vaccine
    - ~70% protection
    - Oral liver-attenuated vaccine, or
    - IM cell-free Vi capsular polysaccharide vaccine

Fungal Infections Associated with Travel

- ➢ Causes / associations
  - o Coccidioides species
  - o Histoplasma sp.
  - o Penicillium marneffei
    - High mortality rate
    - Recurrences
    - Needs treatment for life
  - o More common in HIV infected and immunocompromised persons, esp. Penicillium marneffei contracted in SE Asia and China

Internal Medicine: *Infectious disease*
A. B. R. Thomson

HOSPITAL-ACQUIRED INFECTIONS (HAIS)

> Definition
> - Any infection which develops within 48 hr of hospitalization
> - Absence of evidence that infection was present or incubating pre-hospitalization

- Perform a directed physical examination for fever and infection in a patient in hospital.

Staphylococcus aureus

- Fever often >40⁰C
- Unwell
- Often no specific symptoms/signs

Gram negative septicemia
- Confusion/ delirium often prominent
- Septic shock in 25-40%
- Fever
- Hypotension
- Tachypnea → ARDS

- Often recent (<6 weeks) indwelling line ± local cellulitis

- Endocarditis

- Enter bloodstream

- Occasionally arise from GI tract

- Warm

osteomyelitis

- Usually arise from urinary tract

- Often indwelling urinary catheter

Bacteremia

- Positive blood cultures + no/ trivial symptoms

- Joint infection

- Death rate 20-40%

Adapted from: Davey P. *Wiley-Blackwell* 2006, page 68.

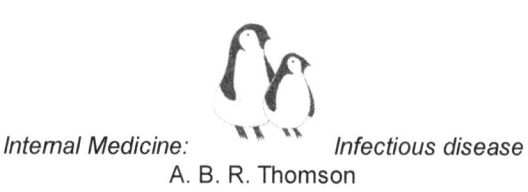

➢ Types

• Give 5 types of HAIs.
  o AAD (antibiotic-associated diarrhea, including C. difficile
  o CAUTI (catheter-associated urinary tract infection)
  o CLABSI (central time-associated bloodstream infection)
  o HAI-MDRO (hospital-acquired infection with multi-drug resistant organisms)
  o HAP (hospital-acquired pneumonia)
  o SSIs (surgical site infections)
  o VAP (ventilator-acquired pneumonia)

Hospital-acquired pneumonia (HAP)

➢ Definitions
  o HAP
    – Symptoms of pneumonia plus new / progressive infiltration on chest X-ray ≥ 48 hr after hospitalization
  o VAP
    – A subset of HAP, occurring > 48 after endotracheal intubation
  o May be caused by MDRO (multi-drug-resistant organisms)
  o Most cases of HAP in the ICU are VAP (ventilator-acquired pneumonia)

➢ Risk factors

• Give 10 factors which ↑ risk of HAP / VAP.

  o Patient
    – Older
    – Fatal disease
    – Trauma
    – Drugs
      ▪ Antibiotics
      ▪ Corticosteroids
      ▪ H2 blockers

  o Lung
    – Ventilation
    – Underlying chronic lung disease
    – Recent large-volume aspiration

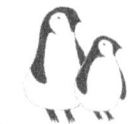

- o Abdomen
  - – Abdominal surgery
  - – NG (nasogastric) tube
  - – Use of H2 blockers

- o CNS
  - – Neurological disease
  - – ↓ LOC (level of consciousness)

- Give 3 factors which ↑ risk of MDRO.

  - o Drugs
    - – Antibiotics
    - – Immune suppression

  - o Hospital
    - – ≥ 5 days hospitalization
    - – Health care-associated exposures

➢ Treatment
  - o Depends upon risk for MDRO (**multi-drug-resistant organisms**)
  - o Risk factors for MDRO
    - – Hospitalization
      - ▪ ≥ 5 days
      - ▪ From a healthcare facility
    - – Drugs (recent)
      - ▪ Antibiotics
      - ▪ Immunosuppressants
  - o No MDRO risks
    - – Ceftriaxone, or
    - – Levofloxacin
  - o MDRO risk
    - – Vancomycin, plus
    - – Cefepime or ceftriaxone

- Give the rational for the antibiotic selection for HAP/VAP associated with risk of MDRO.

  - o Vancomycin – MRSA

  - o Cefepime or ceftriaxone – Pseudomonas aeruginosa

Pearl and Gem
- In CDAAD (Clostridium difficile antibiotic-associated diarrhea) there are presentations other than "diarrhea", including
  - Fever
  - Rectal bleeding
  - Ileus
- CDAAD may develop in the community and in persons not previously exposed to antibiotics

---

HAI-MDRO (Hospital-acquired infections from multi-drug resistant organisms

- Most MDROs are HAI, rather than community-acquired

➤ Causes / associations

- Give the name of 3 common HAI associated with MRDOs.
  - Gram-positive
    - MRSA (methicillin-resistant Staphylococcus aureus
    - VRE (vancomycin-resistant enterococci
  - Gram-negative
    - ESBL (extended-spectrum B-lactamase)-producing Enterobacteriaceae
    - MDR strains of P. aeruginosa

➤ Treatment
- MRSA
  - Vancomycin
  - Linezolid
  - Clindamycin
  - Daptomycin
- VRE
  - Ampicillin
  - Linezolid
  - Daptomycin
- ESBL
- For Carbapenem resistant
  - Carbapeman-sensitive
  - Fluoroquinolones
  - Ertapenem
  - Enterobacteriacease
  - Pseudomonas
  - Acenetobacter
  - Polymycxins
  - Tigecycline
  - Aminoglycosides

CAUTI (catheter-associated urinary tract infection (UTI)

➤ Definition

- ○ Symptoms or signs of UTI in patients with
- ○ ≥ 10^3 cfu (colony forming units) / mL
- ○ ≥ 1 bacterial species in urine sample

Note: In the patient with a urinary catheter, pyuria does not indicate a UTI

➤ Clinical

- ○ If patient with a urinary catheter has UTI symptoms, fever and cultured mental state, suspect CAUTI culture urine, and treat appropriately
- ○ If patient asymptomatic, "don't go looking for trouble" do not do urine cultures o urinalysis.
- ○ If cultures done (inappropriately) in asymptomatic patient with a urinary catheter, do not treat bacterurea or candiduria

➤ Prevention

- ○ Chlorhexidine skin cleaning
- ○ Antibiotic-coated catheters, dressings
- ○ Catheter-care team, e.g. TPN team

➤ Treatment

	Cultures Catheter	Blood	Antibiotic treatment	Catheter removal
○ Colonization	+	-	No	-*
○ Catheter-related bacteremia	+	+	1-3 wk	+/-
○ Complications	+	+	4-6 wk	+

Skin site culture				
○ Exit-site	+	-	1 wk	+/-
○ Tunnel	+	-	1-3 wk	+/-

* Catheter positive, blood culture negative, or transiently positive for coagulase-negative staph' bacteremia
- ○ Antimicrobials – Vancomycin is no MRSA or no

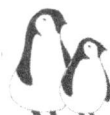

Internal Medicine: *Infectious disease*
A. B. R. Thomson

coagulase-positive Staphylococcus
- Neutropenia or sepsis
- Candidemia
  - Fluconazole
- Candidemia plus sepsis
  - Amphotericin B or echinocandin especially when caused by Candida tropicalis, C. keusei

- Give the indications for performing TEE (transesophageal echocardiography) in a patient with catheter-related infection.

  o Blood cultures positive for S. aureus
  o Signs of endocarditis, such as new murmur

Surgical site infections (SSIs)

- Give the pre- and intraoperative measures which are useful to ↓ risk of SSIs (surgical site infection)

o Preoperative	– Hair	• Clean but do not shave
	– Skin	• Chlorhexidine cleaning solution
	– Lungs	• Supplement O_2
	– Operating room	• Only necessary or staff • Checklist use for compliance to quality improvement procedures
o Intraoperative-antibiotics	– Antibiotics	• Vancomycin and fluoquinolone • Start 1-2 h before surgical incision • Repeat as needed during long procedure • Stop antibiotics within 24 h

CARE OF THE ELDERLY

- Take a directed history for functional assessment in the elderly.

➢ Activities of daily living (ADL)
  o Transfers out of bed
  o Going to the toilet
  o Eating
  o Dressing
  o Getting around the home
  o Bathing
  o Food preparation
  o Stairs
  o Walking

Lifestyle issues

- Take a directed history of lifestyle issue.

➢ **HPI – L DOCC SPARC CIP**
  o **L**ocation
    - Where is the chief complaint experienced?
  o **D**uration
    - How long does the chief complaint last?
  o **O**nset
    - When did the chief complaint start?
  o **C**ourse
    - What are the changes in the chief complaint over time?
  o **C**haracter
    - Describe the quantity and quality of the chief complaint
  o **S**everity
    - Grade the chief complaint on a scale from 0 (no pain) to 10 (worst pain the patient can image) both for its time of onset and the present
  o **P**alliating/ provoking
    - What makes the chief complaint better and worse?
  o **A**ssociated S&S
    - What are the signs and symptoms presenting as a complex with the chief complaint?
  o **R**isk factors
    - What are the factors known to enhance chances of having the chief complaint?

- o Constitutional signs
  - Fever, chills, night sweats, changes in sleep, energy level, weight, and appetite
- o Causation
  - What does the patient think the cause is?
- o Impact on the patient
  - How has the illness affected the patient?
- o Patient's action
  - What has the patient done for the complaint (s)?

- ➤ **PMH- SHIAMS**
  - o **S**urgeries
    - Type, when, outcome (s)
  - o **H**ospitalizations
    - Condition, when hospitalized, outcome (s)
  - o **I**llnesses
    - In adults, always ask about HTN, DM, Hx of cancer, as well as duration and treatments
  - o **A**llergies
    - Drugs, descriptions of reaction (s), MedAlert? EpiPen?
  - o **M**edications
    - Types and dosing
  - o **S**ins
    - Smoking/ alcohol/ drug use
- ➤ Family history
- ➤ Causes / associations
- ➤ Complications

Abbreviations: HPI, history of present illness; PMH, past medical history

Source: Jugovic PJ, et al. *Saunders/ Elsevier* 2004, pages 5 to 9.

Reasons for Falls in Seniors
- ➤ Physiologic
  - o ↓ visual acuity
  - o ↓ night vision
  - o ↓ sensory awareness, touch
  - o ↑ body sway, ↓ righting mechanisms
- ➤ Pathologic
  - o Cardiac
    - Myocardial infarction
    - Orthostatic hypotension

Internal Medicine: *Infectious disease*
A. B. R. Thomson

- o Neurological
  - - Stroke
  - - TIA
  - - Dementia
  - - Parkinsons disease

- o Metabolic
  - - Hypoglycemia
  - - Anemia
  - - Dehydration

- o MSK
  - - Arthritis
  - - Muscle weakness

- o Drug induced
  - - Diuretics
  - - Antihypertensives
  - - Sedatives
  - - Analgesics

Abbreviations: MSK, musculoskeletal; TIA, transient ischemic attack

Adapted from: Jugovic PJ, et al. *Saunders/ Elsevier* 2004, page 35.

Grief and Abuse

- o The classic stages of grief
  - - Patient attempts to limit awareness of condition (shock, denial, and isolation)
  - - Patient has awareness and emotional release
  - - Patient experiences depression
    - ▪ Accepts the reality of loss
    - ▪ Work through the pain of grief
  - - Patient has acceptance and resolution
    - ▪ Adjust to life without the deceased

- o **Feelings** that many grieving people experience.
  - - Anger
  - - Hopelessness
  - - Guilt
  - - Worthlessness

Source: Jugovic PJ, et al. *Saunders/ Elsevier* 2004, pages 196, 198 and 199.

Internal Medicine: *Infectious disease*
A. B. R. Thomson

WOMEN'S HEALTH

Breast Cancer

- ➢ Therapy
  - ○ Surgery
    - – Lumpectomy plus radiation
      - ▪ Tumor < 5 cm
      - ▪ Localized in situ duct carcinoma
    - – Mastectomy
      - ▪ Tumor > 5 cm
      - ▪ Previous radiation therapy
    - – Dissection of axillary nodes
      - ▪ Only if sentinel node is positive
    - – Mastectomy plus radiation
      - ▪ Close surgical margin
      - ▪ Involvement of skin
      - ▪ ≥ 4 axillary nodes

  - ○ Pharmaceuticals, after lumpectomy plus radiation
    - – ER / PR – positive tumor
      - ▪ Premenopausal
        - – Tamoxifen
      - ▪ Postmenopausal
        - – Aromatase inhibitors
          - ▪ Letrozole
          - ▪ Anastrozole
          - ▪ Emaestane
      - ▪ Bone metastasis, or small, asymptomatic visceral metastases
        - – Serial tamoxifen; aromatase inhibitors
        - – Fulvestrant, and
        - – Megrestrol acetate
    - – ER / PR-negative tumors, or endocrine resistant
      - ▪ Sequential single agent chemotherapy, or
      - ▪ Combination chemotherapy
    - – HER2-positve tumor
      - ▪ Trastuzumab ± chemotherapy adjuvant therapy
    - – Adjuvant chemotherapy
      - ▪ Tumor > 1 cm
      - ▪ Any lymph node involvement
    - – Lytic bone disease
      - ▪ Bisphosphonates
      - ▪ Denosumab
      - ▪ Radiation

- Give the reason why women with HER-2 positive breast cancer are given adjunctive therapy with trastuzumab, without anthracycline agents.
  - These agents are cardiotoxic and may impair LV / left ventricular function) and lead to HF (heart failure)
  - Assessment of cardiac LV function is recommended **before** trastuzumab adjuvant therapy for HER2-positve breast cancer

- Prevention
  - If the Gail model predicts that a 35 to 60 year old woman's 5 yr risk of breast cancer is ≥ 1.66%, then tamoxifen or raloxifene may be offered, taking into account the recipient's ↑ risk of
    - TED (thromboembolic disease)
    - Endometrial cancer
  - Tamoxifen and raloxifene reduce the risk of a woman developing breast cancer, but in some women the risk of her developing breast cancer is so high that prophylactic bilateral mastectomy and oophorectomy may be recommended.

- Give 3 factors which should lead to a discussion about prophylactic bilateral mastectomy and oophorectomy
  - Mutation
    - BRCA1 or BRCA2 gene
    - p53 gene
  - Family history
    - 1st degree relative
    - 2nd degree relatives on ovarian cancer the same side of the family   Breast or

Cervical Cancer

Stage

IA1	
– Child-bearing desired	• Loop electrosurgical excision • Cervical conisation
– Child-bearing not desired	• Hysterectomy
II, III, IV	• Radiation • Chemotherapy, cisplatin
Metastatic disease	• Local radiation • Chemotherapy

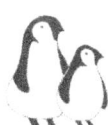

Internal Medicine: *Infectious disease*
A. B. R. Thomson

Disappointing

- o Unlike cervical cancer, screening for endometrial cancer does not ↓ mortality
- o It is not yet established that screening for ovarian cancer ↓ mortality

MEN'S HEATH

Prostate Cancer

- A man presents with acute urinary retention, and a prostate cancer is suspected. The PSA (prostate specific antigen) concentration is increased. Give the next step for his assessment.

    - o Relieve the obstruction and repeat the PSA
    - o Any cause of urinary retention will increase the PSA concentration.

- ➢ Treatment options
    - o Radical prostatectomy
    - o Radiation
    - o Radiation plus androgen deprivation therapy with gonadotropin-releasing hormone agonist (hormonal therapy)
    - o Hormonal therapy
    - o Docetaxel

"Don't worry about the neurobiological mechanisms of motivated learning – just provide a safe, stimulating and welcoming environment."

Grandad

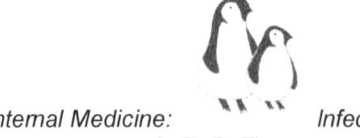

SEXUAL ABUSE ACCOMMODATION SYNDROME

- o Experienced by people who have suffered sexual abuse as children may experience
- o Secrecy and silence
- o Helplessness and vulnerability
- o Entrapment and accommodation
- o Delayed, conflicted, and unconvincing disclosure
- o Retraction

Source: Jugovic PJ, et al. *Saunders/ Elsevier* 2004, pages 86 to 88.

- For an excellent background of:

  ➢ A directed history for physical abuse, please see: Jugovic P.J., et al. *Saunders/ Elsevier* 2004, pages 73 and 74.

  ➢ A directed history for sexual abuse, please see: Jugovic P.J., et al. *Saunders/ Elsevier*, 2004, pages 86 and 87.

  ➢ Reasons why the abused often fail to speak out about their mistreatment and kinds of elder abuse, please see: Jugovic PJ, et al. *Saunders/ Elsevier* 2004, page 209.

SO YOU WANT TO BE A GOOD GENERAL PHYSICIAN!

- You say that the patient "looks his/her stated age. But what conditions make you look older or younger that you actually are?

  ➢ Looks older
    - o Smoking
    - o Drinking in excess
    - o Sunlight in excess
    - o Chronic illness/cancer
    - o Progeria (pathological acceleration of aging)

  ➢ Look younger
    - o Hypogonadism
    - o Panhypopituitarism
    - o You wish!

Adapted from: Mangione S. *Hanley & Belfus* 2000, page 11.

- For an excellent background of how to

> Take a directed history for HIV disease in a man having sex with men (MSM), see: Jugovic PJ, et al. *Saunders/Elsevier*, 2004, pages 45 and 46.

> Take a focused history for Gay and Lesbian health issues, see: Jugovic PJ, et al. *Saunders/Elsevier* 2004, pages 40 and 41.

JUST A FEW OF THE DRUGS TO AVOID IN PREGNANCY-TERATOGENIC

- o Certain
  - – Coumadin
  - – Methotrexate
  - – Misoprostol
  - – Thalidomide

- o Possible
  - – Diazepam
  - – Fluconazole
  - – Statins

Diav-Citrin O and Koren G. Appendix II. In: Therapeutic Choices. Grey J, Ed. 6th Edition, *Canadian Pharmacists Association*: Otttawa, 2011, page 1722-4.

Warning

Use of alcohol in any amounts is **not** compatible with pregnancy or breastfeeding.

"We need to move forward our decisions:
we must operationalize."

Grandad

Internal Medicine: *Infectious disease*
A. B. R. Thomson

TOXIC SYNDROMES FROM DRUG OVERDOSE

- Perform a focused physical examination to determine the cause of drug toxicity.

	Sym	Chol	Anti-Chol	Opioids
o Eyes	Mydriasis	Myosis	Mydriasis	Miosis
o CNS activity	↑	↓	↑	↑
o Secretions				
– Tears	↓	↑	↓	
– Salivation	↓	↑	↓	
– Bronchorrhea	↓	↑	↓	
– Sweating	↑	↓	↑	
o Heart				
– HR	↑	↓	↑	↓
– ↑ BP	↑		↑	↓
– RR	↑		↑	↓
– Temp	↑		↑	
o GU				
– Urination		↑		
o GI				
– Defection		↑		
– Vomiting		+		

Abbreviations: anti-chol, anti-cholinesterases; BP, blood pressure; Chol, cholinesterases; HR, heart rate; RR, respiratory rate; Sym, sympatheticomimetics; Temp, temperature

ONLINE RESOURCES:

- MedEdPORTAL: https://www.mededportal.org/
- Portal of online geriatric education: http://www.pogoe.org/
- AGA educator resources: http://www.gastro.org/gi-fellowship/educator-resources
- http://www.gastro.org/practive/medical-osition-statements
- Home parenteral Nutrition: www.oley.org
- Intestinal transplantation: http://www.intestinaltransplant.org
- CCFA: http://www.ccfa.org
- CCFC (Crohn's and Colitis Foundation of Canada): www.ccfc.ca
- http://www.pathology.pitt.edu/lectures/gi
- www.orl.cz/ehorroby/ustni/vestibulum/veozena
- http://www.pathologyatlas.com
- http://www.mayoclinic.org/gi-risk/mayomodel2.html
- http://mayoclini.org/meld/mayomodel6.html
- www.gastro.org/practice/meicacl-osition-statements
- Natural Comprehensive Cancer Network (NCCN) guidelines: www.nccn.org
- http://www.accessdata.fda.gov/drugsatfda_docs/label/2011/201917lbl.pdf
- http://www.accessdata.fda.gov/drugsatfda_docs/label/2011/201917lbl.pdf
- http://www.aidsinfo.nih.gov/guidelines/
- http://www.fda.gov/Drugs/DrugSafety/ucm291119.htm
- http://www.fda.gov/Drugs/DrugSafety/ucm291119.htm
- http://www.fda.gov/NewsEvents/Newsroom/PressAnnouncements/ucm256299.htm
- http://www.fda.gov/Safety/MedWatch/SafetyInformation/SafetyAlertsforHumanMedicalProducts/ucm291144.htm
- http://www.fda.gov/Safety/MedWatch/SafetyInformation/SafetyAlertsforHumanMedicalProducts/ucm211796.htm
- www.aasid.org/practiceguidelines/Page/default.aspx
- http://www.accessdata.fda.gov/drugsatfda_does/label/2011/201917lbl.pdf
- www.aasld.org/practiceguidelines/Page/default.aspx

Internal Medicine: *Infectious diseases*
A. B. R. Thomson

- National Endoscopy Program : www.grs.nhs.uk
- *MELD, Model for End-Stage Liver Disease, available online calculator: www.mayoclinic.org/meld/mayomodel7.html
- www.motherisk.org/women/index.jsp
- National Endoscopy Program : www.grs.nhs.uk
- CAPstone: http://www.giandhepatology.com
- MedicineNet: www.medicinenet.com/irritable_bowel_syndrome/article.htm
- IBS Support group: www.ibsgroup.org
- UpdateToDate: www.uptodate.com/patients/index
- International Association for the Study of Obesity: http://www.iaso.org
- Liver and intrahepatic bile ducts. www.PathologyOutlines.com
- Medical council of Canada. Weight Gain/Obesity. http://mcc.ca/Objectives_Online/
- Medical Council of Canada. Weight Loss/ Eating Disorders/ Anorexia http://mcc.ca/Objectives_Online/
- Medical council of Canada. Weight loss/Eating Disorders/Anorexia. http://mcc.ca/Objectives_Online/
- http://www.fda.gov/Drugs/DrugSafety/PostmarketDrugSafetyInformationforPatientsandProviders/ucm213038.htm.
- Me'decins San Frontieres: http://www.msf.org
- Recommendations about chemoprophylaxis for malaria. Also see http://www.nc.cdc.gov/travel/yellowbook/2012/chapter-3-infectious-disease-related-to-travel/malaria.htm

INDEX

Note: Page number followed by f and t indicates figure and table respectively.

Internal Medicine: *Infectious disease*
A. B. R. Thomson

Botulism, 56–57
  causes/associations, 56
  clinical, 57
  diagnosis, 57
  treatment, 57
Breast cancer, 73–74
Brucellosis, 59–60
  cause, 59
  clinical, 59
  diagnosis, 60
  treatment, 60

C
CA-MRSA. *See* Community-associated methicillin-resistant *Staphylococcus aureus*
Care of elderly, 70
Catheter-associated urinary tract infection (CAUTI), 68–69
  clinical, 68
  definition, 68
  prevention, 68
  treatment, 69–70, 69t
Cat scratch disease, 3
CAUTI. *See* Catheter-associated urinary tract infection
Cervical cancer, 74–75
Chancroid, 35
Chickenpox, 12–13, 12f
Chlamydia trachomatis, 30–31
  clinical, 30
  complications in women, 30
  demography, 30
  diagnosis, 30
  treatment, 31
Chronic HIV infection, 28–29
Class A bioterrorism agents, 54–57
  anthrax, 54–55
    clinical, 54
    definition, 54
    prophylaxis, 55
  botulism, 56–57
    causes/associations, 56
    clinical, 57
    diagnosis, 57
    treatment, 57
  plague, 56
  small pox (variola), 55, 55t

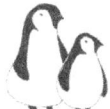

Internal Medicine: *Infectious disease*
A. B. R. Thomson

Internal Medicine: *Infectious disease*
A. B. R. Thomson